Petticoat Surgeon

*This is a volume
in the Arno Press Collection*

SIGNAL LIVES
Autobiographies
of American Women

Advisory Editors

Annette Baxter
Leon Stein
Barbara Welter

*See last page of this volume
for a complete list of titles.*

Petticoat Surgeon

BERTHA VAN HOOSEN

ARNO PRESS
A New York Times Company
New York • 1980

Editorial Supervision: **RITA LAWN**

Reprint Edition 1980 by Arno Press Inc.

SIGNAL LIVES: Autobiographies of American Women
ISBN for complete set: 0-405-12815-0
See last page of this volume for titles.

Manufactured in the United States of America

Library of Congress Cataloging in Publication Data

Van Hoosen, Bertha, 1863-
  Petticoat surgeon.

  (Signal lives)
  Reprint of the ed. published by Pellegrini & Cudahy, Chicago.
    1. Van Hoosen, Bertha, 1863-   2. Gynecologists--Illinois--Biography. 3. Obstetricians--Illinois--Biography. 4. Surgeons--Illinois--Biography. 5. Women surgeons--Illinois--Biography. I. Title. II. Series.
RG76.V36A33 1980   618'.092'4 [B]   79-8820
ISBN 0-405-12864-9

PETTICOAT SURGEON

Petticoat Surgeon

by BERTHA VAN HOOSEN

FOREWORD BY DR. A. E. HERTZLER
author of HORSE AND BUGGY DOCTOR

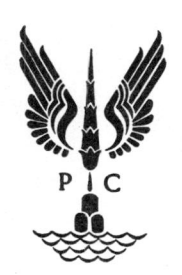

PELLEGRINI & CUDAHY · CHICAGO

Copyright 1947, by BERTHA VAN HOOSEN. All Rights Reserved.

Printed and bound by The Cuneo Press, Chicago, U.S.A.

to ALICE and SARAH

TABLE OF CONTENTS

1. "She-Boy-Agen!" — 3
2. Cackling Chromosomes — 9
3. A 400-Acre Playground — 17
4. A Backyard Kindergarten — 26
5. The Hickory Stick — 35
6. Hayseed Goes to Town — 41
7. Invitation to Medicine — 51
8. "I Swear by Apollo. . . ." — 65
9. Four Years with Obstetrics, Insanity and Surgery — 75
10. A Home Delivery — 94
11. Subjects Not Taught in Medical School — 105
12. A Woman Surgeon's Armageddon — 123
13. The Beginnings of Sex Education — 154

14.	EUROPE AND NORTH AFRICA	167
15.	COOK COUNTY HOSPITAL	182
16.	HEAD OF OBSTETRICS	193
17.	MEDICAL WOMEN ORGANIZE	200
18.	THE GENUS: HEN MEDIC	216
19.	CHINA VIA THE CORAL SEA	235
20.	JAPAN: CAUGHT IN THE 1923 EARTHQUAKE	263
21.	REPORTS ON TWILIGHT SLEEP AND MENTAL HYGIENE	274
22.	MURDER?	287
23.	SHANGRI-LA	307
24.	GREAT GRANDFATHER LIVES	315

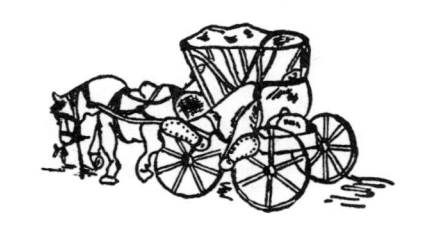

FOREWORD

Dear Girl—

Your publisher is exactly right in saying that a Foreword to your book is unnecessary. Only a conceited self-styled artist would think of painting the lily.

However, I did look you up in Who's Who, and after reading about your accomplishments what little courage I had was dispelled.

All I can say is that you have shown that a woman can achieve first rank in surgery. That is obvious.

If anything could be added to this statement it would be that the manifest need just now is for more women surgeons. I am convinced of this because male operators have made such a terrible botch of pelvic surgery that only women surgeons can bring it back to conservative standards.

You have ridden to distinction on your own momentum. Nobody can add to it.

Very sincerely,
A. E. HERTZLER

PETTICOAT SURGEON

1

"SHE-BOY-AGEN!"

"HI, JOSH! She-boy-agen!" This jocose salutation poured from the grocery store, the blacksmith shop and the grist mill, and reverberated through the hills that encircle the little village of Stony Creek, Michigan. It was intended to frustrate my father who had just been informed that he had begotten a second daughter instead of a long-planned and much-wished-for son.

Eight busy years had passed since Mother had her first baby, my sister Alice. The village gossips, not all women, agreed that Joshua and Sarah were either just lucky or very clever so long to have evaded the common practice of biennial births. In fact, when Mother began to grow big in the belly, her increasing girth was attributed to middle-aged plumpness. Mother was so tight-lipped about her private life as well as about the affairs of her neighbors, that my birth came as a complete surprise to the community.

In 1863, we had two good physicians in Rochester, Michigan, the small town a mile and a half from Stony Creek. They were twins, Jerry and Jesse Wilson, born and educated in Canada, and they appeared on all occasions in long frock coats and high, silk, plug hats. Jesse was married; Jerry, a bachelor.

All night Mother endured the discomfort of labor pains, not even disturbing the hired girl until, in the early morning, it became imperative to send for medical aid. In a fit of imagined modesty she asked for the married doctor. He was out and the unmarried twin, peeved at her preference for his brother, would not come without an urgent invitation.

When he arrived at the story-and-a-half, four-room cottage, he climbed the steep, enclosed stairs and safely deposited his shining stovepipe. In the meantime, I was personally announcing my arrival and the doctor, peering over the top of the lifted sheet, saw me between my mother's outstretched legs, kicking at my placenta, aimlessly waving my fists and howling, as I have many times since, at the unfitness of the male midwife.

I had other reasons for crying: my country was at war—fierce, cruel, civil war. During my first year I was never known to smile, although since then smiling has been one of my distinctive features and displayed at the ghost of an opportunity.

I should, however, have been born laughing instead of crying, for I was that most fortunate of creatures, a wanted baby. I did not have to dimple and dance my way into the hearts of the family. In fact, my birth was regarded as a jubilee to celebrate the liquidation of the farm mortgage, a consummation of Father's ambition to be a debt-free Dutchman.

Nor were my parents the only ones made happy by my entrance into the family circle; my sister Alice was delirious with joy. After she had married and had a baby of her own, she surprised me by relating at a little gathering of women where each one was recalling the happiest moment in her life, "It was when I was told that I had a baby sister. It is so vivid that it seems like an incident of yesterday. I rushed to tell Grandmother who lived around the corner and as I ran over a pile of chips I could feel nothing under my feet but air."

I am more grateful to my mother for catching my father for her husband, than I am for anything she ever did for me, including my birth. For it is to my father that I am indebted for a lucky start in life—I was a jubilee baby. To be a jubilee baby meant being rocked to sleep in the arms of my mother, ridden a la cock horse on Father's strong hide boots, danced and tossed from the arms of one hired man into those of another, cuddled and trundled about by an adoring sister. As a result, I by-passed the dirty, wormlike stage of creeping and crawling. Walking unaided at the age of eight months, I began my eighty year marathon.

Another precious birthday gift was being a breast-fed baby. To be born with a silver spoon in one's mouth does not always insure health or perfect development, but to be born with a mammilla in one's mouth takes out for the baby an irrevocable life insurance. Breast milk, the amount and composition of which changes miraculously from month to month according to the needs of the nursling, gives the baby an immunization through years of protective vaccines acquired by the mother, which no other food can provide. In my own case, immunization through breast-milk must have been perfect, for up to the age of ten I had had none of the diseases of childhood nor any other contageous disease. At the time I was born, during the Civil War, it was a frown of fortune if a baby had to be artificially fed. Even if a child so fed survived the first year, the second summer presented far greater hazards.

I was not only breast-fed, but left to Mother and me I might still be nursing. She was not copying the customs of the mothers of Japan or Labrador, who often nurse their offspring for four or five years. Her sole motive was to make me happy. My weaning was not accomplished through shrieking hunger and physical privation, but by a powerful bribe, a price offered by my Aunt Julia.

Aunt Julia was a lover of finicalities, a milliner by trade, and as the youngest in her family she had been the favored one. She used to visit us on the farm and bring with her some of her town friends. They would go on picnics, play croquet or sit on the long cool porch while Mother cooked delicious meals for them or washed dishes. One day, Aunt Julia appeared in Mother's best dress and asked in a depreciating tone, "Do you think this is all right for the picnic?" "That's Mother's best dress," I screamed, "Mother, don't let her wear it to the picnic." Arching her heavy black eyebrows, Mother looked at me and gave her little laugh of finality. Nothing more was said.

On one of these visits my childless aunt caught me nursing. I stood by Mother's side as she sat in the "Grandma" chair with its ladder back and low flag-bottomed seat scarcely a foot above the floor. Great-grandmother had occupied this chair when she came in the covered wagon from New York State to the Territory of Michigan. A very handy piece of furniture for a nursing more-than-three-year-old little girl.

Aunt Julia made no effort to conceal her disapproval. She could not have been more disgusted if she found me sucking one of Father's pipes. "I think it is horrid for such a big girl as you to be nursing like a little baby. If you will give it up I will bring you a china cup from Mt. Clemens where I am going today."

With anticipatory speed I agreed, and she brought me a china cup decorated with flowers and an inscription. Mother filled it with milk and I ran to my favorite play spot—a pile of stones, the remains of the first log cabin that Great-grandfather built and in which Mother was born.

However, my joy was brief, for only a few delicious possessive moments elapsed before the cup was broken to bits. Bearing the shattered china in both hands I burst into the room where Mother was chatting with some of the neighbors who often dropped in. My wail, "I broke my cup and now I want my titty," was greeted with such deafening laughter that I retired. Never again did I nurse and I boast arrogantly that, if not self-made, I am a self-weaned woman.

GREAT-GRANDFATHER'S GRACE

A story about Rev. Lemuel Taylor

GREAT-GRANDFATHER never liked cornmeal mush, and when he was sparking a girl named Sally, back in New York, he used to come Sunday nights and stay for supper. Sally's father was a Whig and did not care for the Taylors because they were Tories and had fought valiantly for the King.

One Sunday, when Great-grandfather came to call, Sally's father ordered mush and milk for supper to show his disapproval. Just as the family were about to be seated, another suitor appeared who was more pleasing to Sally's family. The mush and milk were taken away at once, and a "company supper" ordered in its place. When they were about to eat, Great-grandfather was asked to say grace. He did, in these words:

> "The Lord be praised, I am amazed
> To see how things have mended
> Shortcake and tea for supper we see,
> Where mush and milk were intended."

2

CACKLING CHROMOSOMES

BORN SPONTANEOUSLY, without medical intervention, and nursed according to my own schedule instead of any pediatric rule, I might be dubbed a fosterling of Pan. I was carefree as that god for sixteen years. Barefooted and bareheaded when weather permitted, I roamed fields that had been the happy hunting grounds of hostile tribes of Indians up to the time when, in 1823, my mother's grandfather, Rev. Lemuel Taylor, bought the land from the government for one dollar and a quarter an acre. President Monroe signed the documents of sale that now, framed, hang in the hall of the old homestead.

Great-grandfather could not have taken seriously the Bible phrase, "the days of his years are three score," for when he was sixty years of age he broke connections with his church and lodge in Aurelius, New York State. Into ox-drawn covered wagons, with ends like Shaker bonnets, looking forward into the sealed future, and backward into the severed past, he packed his lifelong accumulation of worldly goods, and set out on a three months' trek westward, into wild and unsettled country. To remove the temptation of ever returning, he took with him, like a kangaroo with its posterity in its pouch, his wife, his ten children, his six in-laws and his twenty-six grandchildren—sufficient to guarantee a lineage even for a pioneer.

A chromosomic leaning "to go west" may have urged him to begin life at sixty, for his own great-grandfather had sailed from Oxfordshire, England, in the Truelove and landed in Yarmouth, Massachusetts, in 1636, soon after the Mayflower came to Plymouth.

The Erie Canal, "a cent and a half a mile and a mile and a half an hour," was the sole system of transportation in the United States in 1823. It had been completed at that date to within eighty miles of Buffalo. Great-grandfather's family caravan was towed through the Erie Canal to this point, but from there on traveling became more difficult with every mile. Their covered wagons, with bulging loads, were drawn by yoked oxen; and the men, mounted on horses, headed the trek, while the cows and the excited children brought up the rear.

From Buffalo they journeyed around Lake Erie, through Cleveland and Detroit. It was full of pioneers, and the only tavern that would take the Taylor family was so crowded that the eight women and the youngest of their twenty-six children slept in the second story, while the nine men and the older boys had to find places to sleep on the floor in the bar room. Then they went on to Rochester, a few log cabins twenty-five miles north of Detroit. There had been paths, trails, and even roads up to this point, but beyond was unbroken wilderness.

The pioneers now faced the necessity of making a road through virgin forests. They zigzagged, snake-fence fashion, cutting a road among giant trees twenty-four feet in girth, until they reached high ground overlooking a peaceful valley traversed by a noisy creek.

To reach this piece of ground they had for three months jolted over rough roads, with meals poorly cooked or uncooked. They had endured the long comfortless nights, the constant loading and unloading of wagons, and the recurrent embarrassment of ministering to the daily needs of the body. Each discomfort in its own way had helped convert them into tired savages.

As the fagged Taylor family looked into the fertile valley of Stony Creek, their homesick souls became inspired. It was the month of June; the beckoning landscape waved a welcome and begged them to remain.

On the sloping land beside the creek, under the shadow of a circle of high wooded hills, Great-grandfather built a log cabin out of the material at hand. The children brought clay from the creek to fill chinks in the logs and to make the clay mortar for plastering the walls. They constructed a fireplace with a "stick" chimney for heating the house, and a bake oven on the outside for the cooking. Window and door spaces were left open and covered with skins or blankets. In this first log cabin in Stony Creek my mother was born in 1830.

Great-grandfather lived only seven years after coming to the Territory of Michigan, yet that seven-year Taylor saga is a record of accomplishment. He and his sons built the first houses, some grand colonial buildings that are still beautiful, and other houses that, though small and humble, have stood the test of time. They constructed a church, a school, a tavern, stores, smithy shops for shoeing horses, making shoes and turning out wagons—everything contributing to life in an isolated village. Forests were cut down and orchards planted. Thus civilization was pushed farther into the unsettled Northwest.

The Indians, wild animals, inclement weather and privation of pleasures called for the courage of a Daniel, the strength of a Samson, and the steadfastness of the Apostles. There were mosquitoes that called for the patience of Job. These pests were so vicious and numerous that the men had to make a smudge to be able to milk the cows or care for the horses. In addition, there came the miasma from the swamps, and the pioneers shook with ague until cold weather brought relief.

Great-grandfather's conversation carried overtones of the immensity of the natural world which he had conquered and tamed for human living. One of our family anecdotes records the way in which he once threatened to punish one of his grandsons. "Miner, I am sorry to hear of your deviation from rectitude, and if such an abomination ever occurs again, I shall unbutton the sky and let it down on you."

When this man, so rugged, so self-reliant, so even-handed, passed beyond the dominance of his household and his community, it must indeed have seemed as if death had actually unbuttoned the sky, and let it fall, leaving his people groping in darkness.

When young people have every opportunity and advantage in selecting mates, too often marriage is unsuccessful. Yet, among the pioneers who had a Hobson's choice in matrimonial chances, domestic tragedies were rare.

In a family of five girls Mother was kept busy working for some one of her sisters almost all the time; nevertheless, she found ways to attract a jolly young Hollander, Joshua Van Hoosen, who became her wedded husband.

The Van Hoosens migrated to Canada from the Netherlands in 1829, and the following year my father was born in London, Canada, six months before Mother was born in Stony Creek. Poor beyond description, the Van Hoosens moved to Stony Creek with their eleven children when Father was six years old.

Grandmother Van Hoosen worked endlessly and on "almost nothing a year" kept the wolf from the door of her ever-increasing family, but its howling was a constant refrain. Grandfather Van Hoosen never took life seriously. His contribution to the support of his kin depended, in a perverse fashion, upon how much others did. The more they worked the less he exerted himself. Father did not like this hand-to-mouth way of life. He had to pick thorns and sell them to the village woolen mill to earn the money to buy the first pair of shoes for his stone-bruised, chilblain-covered feet. Thorns obtained from hawthorn bushes were used in lieu of pins to close sacks of wool.

When a tad of ten, Father worked in a store that belonged to a sanctimonious deacon of the church. He saw this professed Christian adroitly touch the steelyards with his little finger and make a wide application of his thumb to the yardstick, thereby cheating ever so little in weight and measure. Quite unintentionally this churchman planted the seed that religion was no more than a capacious cloak for iniquity. Father often warned me, "Watch him; he's a Christian."

Father was only fourteen when he determined to be someone, to get ahead instead of living an animal-like existence. One day after hunting, he and his father stopped to rest. Sitting on the top rail of a snake fence Father seized the opportunity for a man-to-man talk.

"Father, if you will buy a farm I will help you pay for it and take care of you and Mother as long as you live, but I must have a deed to the farm. Or perhaps you'd rather I'd pay you $100.00 for my time until I am twenty-one, or else I will run away."

Grandfather scratched his round Dutch head. Well he knew how Father would push the work if they bought a farm. He didn't relish the thought nor did he wish his fourteen year old son to run away so he said, "S'posin' you pay me for your time, Joshua."

Father told me this story when we too were sitting on the top rail of a snake fence overlooking the farm that then belonged to my father. To me it seemed the tale of a tax on an embryo—an entrance fee into life. But since then I have learned that it was not an unusual custom. Father looked with pride on the transaction as his first and most creditable business venture. It was in this fashion, with only three months of schooling and burdened with a voluntarily assumed debt at a time when wages were pitifully small, that Father entered man's estate.

One of his undertakings was a big contract for splitting rails. The rails were located at a distance from Stony Creek and could be reached only by walking. To make matters worse, the weather was extremely cold and he had to eat a lunch frozen by the cold. However, neither distance nor weather was as hard as the clause in the contract which read: "If the work is not completed by the first of March no wages will be forthcoming." Father finished the job far in advance of the stipulated time.

When he was eighteen he completed payment of the debt he owed his parents for thoughtlessly ushering him into a world of poverty and making his childhood fierce, barren, and independent. That he would not keep his promise was unthinkable, for a Dutchman must be as good as his word.

After payment for his time Father saved money to go to California. Our country was in the grip of the gold fever and it must have spread like a contagious disease to have reached and innoculated so simple a lad in so remote a village.

The overland trip to the gold fields was very difficult and dangerous; hence, Father planned to journey by boat from New York to San Francisco, crossing Nicaragua in wagons. His adventure began as soon as he reached New York City. He was six feet tall, with steel blue eyes, and hair so red that, when I was little, I described him to strangers, "That man with pegenty hair and pegenty whiskers and a pipe in his mouth is my father." Pegenty was my private version of magenta, a popular color and my favorite one. At the cheap hotel where he stopped he was spotted at once as a country bumpkin, and a group of roisterers approached him and suggested drinks and a bit of sight-seeing. Father bashfully declined and timidly retired to his room. To his consternation he discovered that his room key did not fit the lock. Nervous and apprehensive, he could not go to bed. Instead, he twisted the bed clothing into a rope and let himself out through the window. Not until he was in his bunk aboard the boat, with his belly belt well cinched about his waist and his tin trunk under his berth, did he feel safe.

In 1853 he returned from California to Stony Creek with this same belly belt full of gold, and with a gold ring embossed with nuggets that he himself had dug. With the gold he bought out the heirs to the Taylor homestead and farm, and with the unalloyed gold ring married my mother on New Year's Day, 1854.

Mother was more fortunate than Father in many ways. She had attended a school which her grandfather had instituted on coming to Michigan, and had acquired enough education to enable her to teach a district school near Stony Creek. She was a woman of Tory blood and breeding with all of the reserve of an aristocrat. Father could, and usually did, intersperse his conversation with oaths that were humorous, harsh or forcible according to his mood. Mother never used any slang and she never joked, although she would rock with laughter at a good story.

Father, unlike Mother, was vocal and a "good mixer." In their diminutive world, he could be found any evening on the steps of the one grocery store, swapping stories with the men who congregated there. Mother never made even a short call in the village, except when her services might be needed on such occasions as sickness or death provided.

Cooking was one of Mother's accomplishments. Without any recipe she could put together a few ingredients and take from the oven delicious pies, flaky biscuits, big creamy cookies, and that rarity, even in those days, salt-rising bread.

She disliked sewing, but never refused to make Father's trousers, because he insisted he could not buy any that fitted so well or were of the same material as those she made. These trousers were of white linen for summer and waterproof for winter. She also made his shirts. These were always fashioned of white muslin; in fact, I never knew him to wear a colored shirt. He wore paper collars which were changed only when he changed his shirt. He kept them on both day and night (sleeping in them) until he changed the next time.

Mother also knit stockings for the entire family until the introduction of the knitting machine, at which time she announced her intention never to knit another stocking or sock. For fifty years she kept her word with the exception of knitting some silk stockings for her small granddaughter, until the call came for hand-knit socks for World-War-I soldiers. Then she laid aside her books and papers and knit a sock a day without complaint, up to the day of the Armistice.

Mother, responsive, percipient and gracious, and almost primitive in her absorption and satisfaction in her family, had no outside interests. Her understanding and loyalty were so deep she could see no wrong in one of her brood. Her man was spotless! Her children were white-headed! Sacrifice for them brought only joy to her soul.

TORY BLOOD

An instance of Mother's independent character

I WAS NEVER more impressed with Mother's almost royal ability to maintain her individuality than when she attended an important dinner party with her hands as black as ebony. She had been shucking walnuts without taking precautions to put on gloves, and her hands had become stained with the juicy shucks—stains that only time could remove.

The invitation to the dinner was unexpected, but she had not the slightest intention of refusing. She selected a nice pair of white gloves which she did not remove during the dinner or until she was at home. Alice and I were amused, and asked, "What was said about the gloves?"

"Why, nothing," she replied.

I pictured her eating dinner with such dignity that all the ladies, instead of being critical, felt rather uncomfortable that they, too, were not wearing gloves.

3

A FOUR-HUNDRED ACRE PLAYGROUND

OUR FARM in Stony Creek is not just a tract of land devoted to agricultural purposes—it is the solar plexus of the Taylor-Van Hoosen family, a sanctum sanctorum. Here my mother, my sister, my niece and I were born; here I received the rudiments of my education and the groundwork of my physical resistance; here the ashes of my ancestors lie buried.

The debt that I owe the farm overwhelms me when, especially in summer time, I watch the city children as they hurry to the park playgrounds carrying with them little pails and shovels.

I compare the silent artificial cement pool where they wade and splash—a cement pool as foreign to nature as a bathtub or a wash basin—with the purling spring-fed creek that pulses and curves like a life-giving umbilical cord over the length and breadth of the farm.

A creek holds increasing fascination in every season of the year. In the spring it becomes swollen like a thing in heat, spreading over its banks, climbing the rising ground on each side, unmindful of bridges or fences, carrying along with it great boulder-like chunks of ice and fence rails, chicken coops or barrels—everything it meets joins in its mad frolic.

After June, as summer advances, it shrinks to a tiny shimmering brook, now hurrying along, fighting rocks and pebbles, now resting at some sharp bend to make a deep dark pool, roofed by overhanging boughs.

When the fall comes, the rains bring the creek back to a near-river stream, and it flows majestically along byways hung with the crimson and yellow of the maples, the burnished copper of the oak and the dull green of the tamarack and pine.

In winter, through banks rimmed with ice, it glides furtively, now flashing in the sun, now hidden by a bridge of snow.

I knew the place of growing and the time of blooming of all the flowers that veiled the countryside in kaleidoscopic splendor from March till late in fall. On the steep hillside came first the hepaticas, cowslips, adder tongue and blood root—together with the sweet-smelling buds of wild crab apple and the thorny hawthorn. In June, deep in the swampland, under the low-branching tamaracks, blossomed the pitcher plants and pink lady-slippers—exquisite orchids. In July, above the tops of the snake fence, waved the fleecy white umbels of elder that bore first crimson, and later, lustrous purple berries. In August, in swales and by the roadside, spread the gay field lilies and the china red white-root. Through September and October and far into November, over the meadows, grew wild asters and goldenrod in extravagant profusion.

Without any worry over planting, cultivating, or watering, year after year this wild garden provided flowers for me to pick when and in what quantities I wished—flowers to pull to pieces, to throw away, to play with, or to carry to the house and arrange in vases.

After the flowers, with surprising speed, came fruit. Mother was so inordinately fond of fruit that my sister Alice declared she must have been a bird in another incarnation. In this respect I took after Mother. From Father I got my big appetite. He said that he was always hungry and that he had never left the table when he could not have eaten another meal with relish. I understand, for I confess to the same vulgar appetite.

After six long, cold months when there was nothing green available except cabbage (canning vegetables is a twentieth century achievement) I began my wild food menu by eating the crisp wood sorrels with their sharp acid taste; the aromatic sassafras leaves and the soft yellow bark; young wintergreens and their spicy red checkerberries; and sweetflag, a marsh herb with thin inner leaves, long green buds, and pungent roots that I was expert in candying. The mallow, a most persistent weed, has a seed shaped like a miniature green cheese. Mother and Alice would shake with laughter watching my absorption (I was only two years old) in hunting these tidbits and eating all I could find.

The first wild fruit to ripen was the mandrake, resembling a yellow plum. Chokecherries, the wild crab apple, the mealy red thorn apple, and sour wild grapes followed.

After the fruit came the nut season when butternuts, black walnuts, hickory nuts, hazelnuts, beechnuts, and a few chestnuts in privately owned gardens could be gathered. Father owned a twenty-acre wood lot in an adjoining county, and so many walnuts and hickory nuts grew there that we would have been able to market them but for the marauding excursions made every fall by the townspeople in neighboring cities.

Gathering wild flowers and fruit, hunting bird's eggs, and fishing for tadpoles and snails in stagnant pools, kept me climbing trees and wandering up hill and down dale.

Botany and horticulture, as well as ornithology and entomology, were not words in my country vocabulary. Nevertheless, through Alice's instruction, a foundation was laid in those branches of science that proved to be of use in later years. She taught me how to gather, press, dry and preserve the wild flowers for an herbarium; how, by making tiny holes in each end of bird's eggs, to blow out their contents and arrange them in a collection. She provided me with a net to catch, and a cyanide bottle in which to kill, shining beetles and gauzy butterflies that I impaled on a pin so that their beautiful spreading wings might dry. I was so young when I mastered many scientific names that I have never forgotten them. A large aquarium made according to my sister's directions was a delight all through the long winter, for balanced with water plants and snails it afforded daily lessons in biology.

I spent little time in the house and had no conscientious feeling about helping Mother with the housework. I was the doglike companion of my father and, in consequence, acquired an empirical foundation in agronomy and animal husbandry. When Father announced, 'Well, lambing is over and the creek is pretty high so I guess we better shear next week," I trembled with delight. Sheep shearing was a regular spring occurrence. Before shearing, the sheep were washed in the creek, which was deep and wide at that time of year. This annual event reminded me of the outdoor baptismal exercises that took place in the village mill pond as a climax to the winter revival meetings. The fervid injunctions given by the preacher to his flock sounded to me like the shouts of the hired men—"for Christ's sake!" "Jumping Jesus!" and "God Almighty"—as they balanced themselves in the water and washed the sheep "white as snow." Then too, the gasping, ducking converts seemed as averse to the chilly mill pond as the struggling sheep to the cold creek. At baptismal time, Father and I always found a secluded spot overlooking the mill pond, from which we could get a good view of the immersion spectacle, and as we walked slowly home behind the bedraggled neophytes, Father would remark, "Just like my sheep— they're doused in the mill pond, then fleeced good in the church."

Preparatory to shearing, the big barn was fitted out with benches made of planks stretched across saw-horses. Empty haymows were fenced in for the waiting sheep, and the boxing board set up. A group of shearers that went from farm to farm were employed to shear the sheep, but Father and I boxed the wool. The docile sheep lay quiet and frightened while the wool was being removed. When released, they ran, a streak of white, out into the pasture to hunt their lambs that hardly recognized the slim, snowy figures of their mothers. As soon as a sheep was shorn, Father gathered up the gossamer fleece and placed it on the boxing board, made with hinged parts that could be folded into a box form, each part notched and threaded with string to tie the gleaming wool into a small square package. These were weighed, and then I took them to the house to be stored in the parlor, clean and warm, until sold.

When spring planting came, corn was the first crop we put in. Wearing a strong apron, the pockets of which were filled with shelled corn, I dropped several kernels into holes that Father dug and afterwards covered with soil.

At corn-husking time, with my small husking peg made to fit the third finger of my right hand, I husked shock after shock of the yellow corn. Father untied and spread the bundle of corn on the ground, and I husked on one side, he on the other, both on our knees. I was ambitious to meet him half way, or better, to beat him, but his fingers were too nimble.

For potato planting the "spuds" were brought to the woodhouse and cut, with one or two eyes in each piece. I enjoyed the cutting, but even more, driving the horses to the field with the seed potatoes. Filling my little basket with them I dropped several chunks into each hole. The potato crop needed constant attention; hoeing to build up the hills and sprinkling with Paris green to destroy the bugs.

Ploughing, cultivating, and getting in the winter supply of wood were left entirely to the hired men, but Father never allowed them to milk because he could not trust them to strip the cow's udders, for if every drop was not removed, the cow might dry up. I loved to watch Father milk. My hands, even when I used both of them, were too small to coax the milk out of the cow's bag.

At harvest time I trotted behind the mowing machine until weary, and then sat in the fence corner beside the pail of ice water till Father made the round of the field. Unlike Father, many farmers took fermented drinks with such alluring names as cherry bounce, raspberry vinegar, or hard cider to the fields in hot weather. But one of Father's brothers, while walking from Rochester to Stony Creek on a bitterly cold New Year's night, had been so intoxicated that he was overcome by cold, and froze to death. Father was never reconciled. He became a strong prohibitionist and would allow no liquor on the place.

When the farm work was a little slack, we pulled stumps. The farm, when Father bought it from Mother's relatives, was for the most part woodland that had to be cleared before crops could be raised. Pulling stumps was the most absorbing of all jobs. We drove to the field in the lumber wagon drawn by the big team, Jim and Charlie. The wagon was loaded with heavy chains, grappling irons, spades, picks and crowbars.

After we had dug around the stump, chains were fastened to the large roots and the trunk. The horses, hitched to the long chain, were started at a good pace and as soon as the slack in the chain was taken up, they reared and heaved. The chain went taut, but the stump obstinately clung to its hold on the dry earth. Again and again there was readjusting of chains, more digging with shovels, and more prying with the crowbar. Then suddenly the stump would roll over on the ground, and the horses would stop in apparent amazement.

Sometimes we loaded the stump up on the wagon, and took it home to be burned in the big barrel-shaped stove in the dining room. At other times we dragged it to a corner where the snake fence was showing weakness.

One of my earliest lessons in physics occurred when Father installed a water system for the house and barns. In 1865, after my grandmother's death, we moved into the frame house that Grandfather had built in 1840. There were so many gushing springs on the hillside across the creek that Father determined to try to pipe the spring water from the hillside to the house.

To provide pipes to conduct the water, he cut tall tamarack trees, and by boring holes through them from one end to the other, made them into what were known as "pump logs." The next step was to drive the small top-end of one log into the larger bottom-end of another, and to construct in this manner, a sufficient length of pump logs to carry the water from the spring down the hill, tunneling across and under the creek, then up a smaller hill to the house.

While the work was progressing, there were plenty of men looking on, ready to laugh at "Josh's Folly," but Father always met them with, "Water will always seek its level."

When the trial came, the spring water from the hillside came gushing and singing through the buried tamarack logs, to pour forth in a never-ending stream into a big half-barrel just outside the door of Mother's kitchen.

Many times when Father entered the woodhouse, bulging with wood split, corded, and ready to burn, he would stoop and drink a dipper of delicious spring water, remarking, "Your mother is a lucky woman! Wood on her back, and water in her eye."

Mother never seemed to appreciate this ambiguous joke, but it made my father chuckle a long time.

Father soon became interested in extending his waterway, and finally laid enough pump logs to carry the water from the house to a fountain in the dooryard, then to the horse barn, from there to a roadside trough, and on into the cow barn.

The fountain was only a cement basin with the whirling spray of a lawn sprinkler in the center of it, but a fountain in the yard of a farm house attracted much attention, and the place was known all over the county for having this water system, and a fountain. The roadside trough was a long wooden box astride the barnyard fence, one-half on the highway, and the other in the barnyard. This was a favorite place for men from far and near, to stop and water their horses. When Father wasn't busy, he often spent many hours here exchanging ideas, or at least expressing his own, while the horses drank and drank as if they had never tasted such water.

Several years after Father had supplied his family and all our farm animals with pure pine-tanged water, he built a barn. This was my initiation into the science of building. My vocabulary swelled with new words—joists, beams, scaffold, rafter, and many others. But of even greater importance, it was then that I watched the growth of a structure from its foundation to completed cupolas. Father constructed the barn from the trees and stones found on the place, even as Great-grandfather had built the first log cabin in Stony Creek out of native material. The barn was called the "big" barn because it was the largest in the county. Father had made it one hundred and one feet long—in order to exceed the length of another barn that was only one hundred! The basement was of field stones gathered from the pastures and the roadsides, and the framework was of hand-hewn trunks of oak, cut and drawn from the woods during the winter. When all the timbers were ready and the basement laid, the farmers in the community were invited to help put the timbers in place and, quite as important, have dinner with us.

The success of that dinner devolved upon Mother. Seventy-five men were to come and many wives, ostensibly to assist Mother.

Days before the raising we commenced to get ready. There were bushels of potatoes to be pared; bread, pie, and cake to be baked; and several batches of cookies, lest the cake give out. There was meat enough to fill the oven in the kitchen, as well as the one in the woodhouse stove. Coffee was made in the clothes boiler. There were rolls of butter, pitchers of thick cream, pickles and jellies. Preparation had to be made for supper as well as dinner, for many came from a distance and no self-respecting farmer would think of allowing anyone to leave hungry if he could be persuaded to stay.

The woodhouse was put into shape to be used as a washroom for the men. The porcelain basins were taken from the bedroom sets, all the tin basins from the kitchen and barn, together with dishes of Mother's soft soap. These were arranged either in the sink in the woodhouse or on benches just outside the door. Stacks of towels were ready, and dippers with which to dip the spring water from the half barrel.

One interesting feature of the raising was the placing of the cornerstone taken from the ruins of the first Masonic temple that had been built in Michigan, on the top of Mt. Moriah. In a pocket in the cornerstone Father placed his pipe, samples of the current newspapers, and currency.

To celebrate the completion of the barn Father and Mother took a trip to Philadelphia to attend the World's Fair. This was in 1876—a big year for our family—for besides having the new barn and the World's Fair visit to make it memorable, it was the year that Alice entered the University of Michigan, opened to women only six years before.

I was thirteen years old and while Father and Mother were away in Philadelphia I was given full charge of the housekeeping. I cooked the meals, made the butter and did all the work, while Alice, with the assistance of Great-aunt Charlotte, sewed from early morning till late at night to finish numberless tucked, ruffled and embroidered petticoats, corset covers, drawers, and nightgowns to take to college.

One of my shortcomings that even farm training has not corrected, is lack of moderation. On this occasion I sold the butter so short (I was allowed all the butter-money while my parents were away) that Mother on her return was aghast to have to buy butter for the first time in her life.

I learned many things on the farm, but especially how to meet realities. When I wanted playthings, I made them—boats whittled out of scraps of wood—cows, milk pans, and churns cut out of pumpkins—playhouses built of material from old buildings—dolls' dresses and hats made out of odds and ends. When I longed for companions, I made my choice of all the farm animals, the birds and fishes. When I just wanted to run, I had a four-hundred-acre farm for my unrestricted arena. When I wanted to eat, the garden, the cellar, the bushes and brambles, the roots and the gums—all fed me. I was never hungry.

4

A BACKYARD KINDERGARTEN

AS A LANDSCAPE project the backyard is an eyesore, but as a kindergarten engineering laboratory it is without a rival. Backyard activities differ with every day and every season. Each day I made a circuit of the dozen small, backyard buildings that were a vital necessity to farm life.

My first visit was to the backhouse, where there was a small, low seat that had been made especially for me. Through the half-open door I took note of outside happenings while I studied the pictures in the papers that filled a box in one corner. If I loitered long enough, the dishes would be washed and wiped during my absence.

The backhouse afforded a genuine retreat when I sought solitude or was emotionally disturbed. Every month Alice had attacks of severe pain, and on one of these occasions Mother discovered me in the backhouse, where I was hiding and crying my eyes out. "What in the world is the matter?" she asked.

"I am sure she is going to die."

"Nonsense! Go wash your face and stop crying."

Because Mother seemed almost amused at my distress I got the notion that I was an adopted child. I did not look like Mother or Alice. It meant nothing to me that I was the very image of my father. Nell Watson, a neighbor child, also thought that she had been adopted, and that we were blood sisters. Whenever I passed her house, she would lean over the gate, sticking out her head like one of the ganders, and hiss, "Does she treat you all right?"

The "she" was Mother.

"Yep," I answered, and skipped along.

The backhouse was attached to the end of the woodhouse, and Mother wished to have a door cut between the two buildings so that the backhouse could be reached without going out of doors. Mother's plea was that when old ladies visited us, they were unduly exposed if the weather was rainy. Father met this with the pleasing promise, "Don't worry, Sarah. I will beau the ladies with an umbrella whenever they want to go to the backhouse."

Father was actually such a prude and his offer so completely out of character that the argument ended in a big laugh. However, Mother was no amateur in getting her way and soon finagled an indoor toilet out of an outdoor backhouse.

Each one of the backyard buildings had a special interest for me. The icehouse was set over a deep excavation and made of rough lumber with windowless walls and a door packed with sawdust. It was filled with ice as soon as the mill-pond froze over. The men sawed the ice into blocks. These they loaded upon the box of the bobsleigh until it looked like a floating iceberg. Father and I packed the chunks away between layers of hay and topped the whole with sawdust. Few farmers had icehouses.

Soon after the icehouse was filled, Father "went fishing" to Lake St. Clair, twenty miles away, where he bought and brought back a wagon-box load of fine fresh fish of all kinds. These were spread on the top of the ice, and we ate fried fish, mashed potatoes and milk gravy until the fish were gone.

Every day all summer, I inspected the height of the ice, wondering if it would last till cold weather (it always did) and looked over the food stored there for refrigeration.

The smokehouse was constructed of red brick with a dirt floor. Its beams were hung with hams and bacon, and when I opened the door cautiously so as not to let out the smoke, the savory odors made me grunt with delight.

I hunted the hens' eggs every day and when, after circling through the henhouse, I moved on, I left the hens cackling, the roosters crowing, the turkeys gobbling, the geese hissing, and the peacock strutting proudly. Mother gave me one cent a dozen for all the eggs I brought to her, and my allowance depended upon my skill and zeal as a hunter. Even if the egg was addle or cracked, no discount was made.

It was real sport to hunt the eggs in the spring, for the hens, wanting to set, would steal their nests, and before I could find them would appear with a brood of downy chicks. Often I had to crawl on my belly under some of the outhouses, and wiggle back, crab-fashion, with my hands full of eggs. Sometimes I found the nest full of broken shells from which the chicks had just emerged; at other times, through the blood-stained shell, I saw the head of the chick appearing; while from other eggs came a persistent tapping, followed by cracking of the shells.

The corn barn, or corncrib, was a curiously constructed building, with a top much larger than the base. It had sides made of narrow boards with spaces between to prevent the corn from "sweating," and was conveniently near the hogpen. With a couple of ears of corn I could tempt the huge snorting sows to lift their fat bodies out of the deep mud in which they were almost buried and come waddling to the fence.

There was a large revolving grindstone that I never passed without turning its crank rapidly many times to see how long it would run after I had left it. Near it, was an enormous iron kettle that tempted me to run around it until I was out of breath. The big kettle was used for scalding the hogs at hog-killing time and for making soft soap.

A few steps from the kettle was the leach, a tall hod-shaped box set on legs and filled with wood ashes. When water was poured over the ashes it seeped through and trickled out at the bottom as a dark brown liquid, called lye. For weeks Mother saved all the fats possible and, when the soap-making day came, they were boiled with the lye in the iron kettle, and we had barrels of soap with which to fight country dirt.

The study of anatomy, my favorite subject, was begun in the back yard at hog-killing time. After a fire had been made under the big iron kettle that was filled with water, the corn-fattened hog was soused in the boiling water, and then suspended by its hamstrings from a gibbet that had been made out of poles from the woodpile. Knives and axes had been sharpened at the grindstone. As soon as the bristles had been scraped from the hog's skin, leaving it pink and clean, the belly of the hog was expertly slashed from tail to snout with a big knife, and the glistening fat-flecked guts, the purple liver, crimson heart and spongy lungs rolled, a trembling mass, into the big dishpan. Mother and I received them and picked away all the fat, which she melted into lard. Then came the work of the sharp ax, and the huge empty carcass was converted into hams, shoulders, tenderloins, ribs, pigs' feet, hunks of fat for salt pork and pieces for sausage.

Without a peep into Grey's anatomy I reveled in seeing what was under the skin. Hog killing was not the only opportunity to pursue this fascinating study, for I early learned to dress chickens and turkeys—where to cut, and how, without breaking the gall bladder, to remove all the viscera.

Production and reproduction is the rural theme that marks the time and synchronizes everything on a farm. I was enrolled in the kindergarten backyard laboratory for a course in biology, which differs from anatomy in that it is a study of life in action. I was never deceived into believing that I was found under a rosebush, or in a cabbage patch. There was never any clandestine conversation in the family.

A knowledge of sex came to me as early, as gradually and from as natural sources as my teeth and my hair. I cannot remember when I was bald and toothless.

The geese provided an early lesson. Every spring, on account of poor drainage, there was a fair-sized pond in the back yard. In summer this became a mud hole, but at all seasons the pond was a rendezvous for the geese that Mother kept for many years. They were of value for their feathers, but Mother never cooked a goose or a goose's egg though she raised great flocks of them.

Goose-picking day was very exciting, because I was always a little afraid of the hissing, long-necked ganders that Mother grasped fearlessly by their legs, and placed on her lap, breasts upward, their snakelike heads reaching in this and that direction. She would seize handful after handful of feathers, and literally tear them from the breasts of the geese, depositing the fluffy clumps in a big sack. They were then given their freedom and waddled away looking sheepish, no doubt feeling like Nancy Etticoat, whose petticoat had been cut to her knees.

This pond provided a make-believe ocean on which to sail my boats. While manipulating my fleet, I could watch the geese. At times they seemed to be very affectionate, running their bills up and down each others' long necks, until one of the geese would sit down. This was an invitation for her gander lover to mount gracefully upon her back, maintaining his balance by a firm grip on the goose's neck, and then, after a moment's wigwagging of tails, to step off. Both the goose and the gander, stars in this love drama, opened their mouths at this juncture and filled the air with a kind of victory pæan in which the other geese joined.

Another event of absorbing interest was the visit of the stallion. All of our horses were staid and commonplace in comparison with this wonderful animal that came cavorting into the barnyard, with arching neck and flying mane. I had never been told, but I knew that I should not stay at the barn when the stallion was there. However, deeply interested in the stallion, I climbed to the top of the haymow and selected a generous-sized knothole from which, as Peeping Tom, I could satisfy my curiosity. The stallion, unhitched from the sulky, was led into the barnyard to meet the bay mare. When he caught sight of her, he tossed his head, and with prancing gait, ran towards her, but she walked away with averted glance. He whinnied and followed her. This flirtation continued for some time until the man with the stallion looked at his watch, and said, "She won't take him; I'm goin'." Soon the sulky, the man, and the big handsome stallion were flying down the road.

Soon after this, I noticed one of the cows jumping upon the back of another. The hired man also noticed it and said to my father, "I better take that cow away tomorrow." The next day he led the cow to a neighboring farm, and returned with her after dinner. There were many repetitions of this experience, and slowly this jigsaw puzzle grew.

Birth is such an inspiring demonstration of the beginning of life that every young child, long before the age of sexual awakening, should enjoy the ocular evidence of it.

To my pet cat I am indebted for such a valuable opportunity. She was white with blue eyes, and I had trained her to lie on her back in the baby buggy, and let me wheel her around the village square, without her making an attempt to escape. One night I heard howling and spitting, and wanted to go to her rescue, feeling sure that she was being hurt. Mother said, "Don't worry. She'll take care of herself."

Not long after, I noticed that my pet was getting plump, and that every week added to her waistline until she became so distended that she walked with difficulty. One day when the cat was scratching among some clothes lying in a corner, Mother saw her, and seizing a broom, literally swept her out of doors, remarking, "Get out! You can't make a nest in here!"

It interested me that my cat was going to make a nest, and I followed her. She dragged herself from one place to another, finally settling down at the end of the woodpile on one of the rags that Mother had used when she picked geese. This was my golden opportunity. Climbing to the top of the woodpile, opposite the place where the cat had settled herself, I crawled on my hands and knees until I reached a point directly above the cat.

I was none too soon, for as I looked down from my vantage point, I saw a glistening bag protruding from the hind end of the cat, and even as I looked, the bag ruptured, and a tiny, slick kitten-head emerged, followed quickly by the body. The mother cat caught in her mouth a slender, white, fleshy cord that attached her to the kitten, and jerked it so vigorously that it came away from her with a small piece of red meat hanging to it. The mother swallowed this piece of meat, and the kitten, freed, rolled to the ground. The little thing was very wet, but the mother licked it in none too gentle a manner.

I was sorry that I had not more time to study this marvelous spectacle, but my regrets were soon dispersed, for another bag appeared, ruptured, and was followed by the birth of a second kitten. In all there were five, and I watched until the whole brood were working vigorously at the mother's breasts.

To witness spontaneous birth gives a sublimity to life and motherhood, but to come face to face with an impossible delivery leaves only the impression of the terrible price paid and the fruitlessness of the pain endured.

One morning I crossed a part of the barnyard fenced off for animals in trouble. Climbing the snake fence, I cought sight of a sheep lying on the ground. I had seen farm animals under many and various conditions, but nothing comparable to this.

The dead ewe was lying on her side, and protruding from her body was all but the head of a baby lamb. I settled myself on the top rail of the fence, drinking in the mysterious sight.

Thinking I heard footsteps, I rapidly scrambled down from my observation seat and retreated towards the house. It proved to be a false alarm, and I climbed back with breathless haste. I paid no attention to the lapse of time; spellbound, I stayed on and on, my eyes fixed on the luckless ewe.

As the hour for dinner approached, I broke my vigil long enough to go to the house to eat dinner with the family. I found that I could easily slip away after dinner, and returned to the unborn lamb with fresh enthusiasm until supper time.

After supper I tore myself away and planned to return. Alas! The sun had set and it was getting dark; there was nothing to do except go to bed and wait for the morning.

The next morning I dressed hurriedly, and after a perfunctory breakfast, I was back at my post and all was well. Nothing had been disturbed. The entire day was spent in looking, looking, looking, only interrupted by the meals that had to be eaten.

On the following day I found that the dead ewe and her unborn lamb had been removed.

It must have been several years later that the daughter of a neighboring farmer took me aside, and in profound secrecy whispered, "I know something." We had to have the proper environment before she would tell me. When we were hidden in a deep recess in the strawstack, she said, still whispering, "I know where babies come from."

I was disgusted with all of this palaver over what I supposed everybody knew. I got up, disappointed, and walked away, saying, "Who doesn't?"

"How long have you known these things?" she demanded.

I replied, and I believe I was truthful when I said, "I have always known them."

And so it happened that while, unassisted, I was getting an impregnable foundation in sex biology, in my own back yard, most children were being kept in ignorance of sex.

The backyard kindergarten even afforded social training through an annual Christmas tree which was set up in the tool house, and to which I invited all the village children.

Father and Mother never had a Christmas tree for us alone because Father seemed to find a note of dishonesty in the myth of Santa Claus. My presents were given to me at once and never saved up for any special time. With the exception of hanging up my stockings and having oysters and turkey for dinner, Christmas was much the same as any other day. Yet the Santa Claus character gripped my fancy to the extent that when I was very young, I took upon myself the responsibility of assuming that role. Our community Christmas tree was set up in the tool house, furnished with a carpenter's bench, tools, a box woodstove, and apparatus for mending harnesses and repairing wagons and farm implements. Here Mother sorted and weighed goose feathers, shucked walnuts, and stored rags and paper. None of the village children were ever allowed to enter the tool house except on Christmas Day, and this gave a fillip to the party.

My ambition to give at least ten presents to each child kept me working continually from one Christmas to the next. My egg money was not sufficient to buy even one "store" present, so I had to manufacture out of mere nothings one hundred and fifty or two hundred presents. Month after month, all the year round I viewed everything through Santa Claus spectacles that I wore night and day. The rag bag was productive; worn-out stockings supplied bits of yarn; the creek bed was a treasury of shells, bits of broken glass and colored stones. My creative genius was restrained by only one thing—it must be possible to label the present and hang it on the tree.

Mine was a one-man show, for I received no assistance or even a pretense of interest from my family, until the joyous season arrived. Then the hired men searched the woods for a nice evergreen tree, and cut cedar boughs to decorate the walls. These boughs were held in place by tin stars fashioned out of oyster cans, and the tree was wreathed with strings of cranberries and festoons of popcorn. Planks resting on sawhorses furnished seats, and the tree was fastened into the carpenter's bench.

Alice, dressed as Santa, cut the presents from the festive gift-burdened tree and read, one by one, the names of the children who were exploding with Christmas spirit, like corn in a hot popper. After the tree had been relieved of its homemade childish exhibits, Mother appeared—her hair waving softly above her heavy, dark brows, and her stiffly starched calico dress nestling against a fresh apron. With royal dignity she treated the youngsters to sparkling Christmas cider and fresh, plump, golden-brown doughnuts.

During the preschool days that I spent in the backyard kindergarten, I was in a world as peculiarly my own as while I was wiggling in the womb. Every experience that came to me in the busy years that followed had its beginning in those backyard years.

5

THE HICKORY STICK

I AM A PROUD product of the public school system. My copper-colored locks had been twisted into soft curls when Mother led me up the lane that cuts the village square in two and left me in the Stony Creek rural school like a lump of unworked clay in the hands of the potter. Twenty years passed before that mass was finally shaped into the form of a woman doctor. That it ever became so molded is to the credit of the free schools that were always open whenever I was ready to enter.

Father did not expect or desire his daughters to be precocious, but there was such a marked difference in our mental molds that he became concerned about me. When I was five years old, I knew only a few of the letters of the alphabet. At that age, Alice had been able to read any chapter in the Bible. When she could scarcely toddle, she would follow Mother with a book, asking her the names of the letters and then the words, till she could read.

Before I was a year old I had earned the nickname, Ginger, because of my hot, quick temper. When it was noised about the village that Josh's Ginger didn't know her letters, the family pride was touched.

In an attempt to teach me, Father laid the Rural New Yorker across his knees and called, "Come, Bertha, let's see if you can tell me some of these letters."

I stood, very serious, in front of him, and gazed with feigned interest at the rustic letters of the newspaper's title before me.

"What is that?" Father asked, pointing to the letter O.

I knew that one.

Father tried another, an easy one.

I knew that, too.

When he pointed to the letter E, it looked very queer and perfectly unfamiliar—the more I looked at it the surer I was that I had never seen it before. Then, as I have often done in a dilemma, I made a joke. Crumpling the newspaper in my small hands, I rushed away, calling to Father, "Boogerman! Boogerman!"

He ran after me as I had expected, and the lesson ended in a wild game of tag. Father sighed and looking at Mother, said, "I am afraid she is going to be like old—," and he named the village moron.

It never occurred to anyone that I might have been interested in learning words instead of ABCs, as children nowadays are taught. No one seemed to think that I might be unconsciously progressive.

The district school was an ungraded, one-teacher-for-all institution and was considered "good enough for farmers." In this school I not only recited my own lessons, but every day I heard all of the other children recite theirs. As a result I learned rapidly, and at the age of ten was more advanced than children of a corresponding age in the town school in nearby Rochester.

Although school teaching was one of the few occupations open to women in the nineteenth century, I had but one woman teacher in the score of years that I spent in school. In the Stony Creek school a man teacher was always employed on the grounds that it was necessary to have a teacher physically able to punish the large boys. Having seen no corporal punishment (Father never allowed even the animals to be whipped), many times I grew faint watching the teacher snatch a hulking farm boy by the coat collar, swing him out of his seat to his knees in the center of the room, and with a strong leather strap belabor him till he regained his feet, only to be thrown on his knees again and again.

The girls were never flogged, but they were punished by being forced to extend a hand while a ferule was bought down upon it until they no longer drew the hand away.

Everything was open and above board in our family, yet like most young people, I reveled in secrets. Someone in school always had a secret to trade. Of all secrets none offered so much sport as a game in which a small group of girls of my age indulged. The Bible was a much revered book, and we were taught that every word in it was golden. Imagine our feelings when we discovered in the Bible a nasty word that everybody said no nice person would use. On this basis we invented a contest in which the one who could find the greatest number of these taboo words was the best man. These were good old Anglo-Saxon words that have been expurgated from modern Bibles. What tickled us most of all was to see how pleased our teacher or our parents were when they found us thumbing over the leaves of the Bible. It saved us from having to set the table, fill the wood box or even to let the dog out. I envisioned how Mother would lift her arching black eyebrows if she knew that the little marks I was making on a bit of paper only meant that I had found another word—an awfully dirty word.

Although I spent thirty hours every week in the schoolroom, we were never given any "homework" and that left almost twice as much time to devote to farm activities. As soon as I got out of school I peeled off my school dress and apron, put on very old clothes and ran like a deer from one point of interest to another. On Saturday nights I took a bath in the big wooden washtub filled with water heated in a wash boiler on the kitchen stove. On Sundays we slept an hour later than on weekdays, and I often dressed before dinner in my much beruffled white muslin dress with a blue sash, my leghorn hat with blue streamers, and my blue kid shoes. I was very proud, almost too proud, of some of my wearing apparel. My bright blue kid shoes thrilled me with their beauty. I openly expressed such satisfaction in them that Father reproved me and said, "I don't think you should be so proud of your shoes."

"How can I help it when they are so pretty?"

Once in all my Sunday best I set out after dinner to walk to the graveyard, but thoughtfully took the butterfly net and bottle lest I should see some fine specimen, and not be prepared to catch it.

Sure enough, just before I reached the bridge over the creek, on the way to the burial ground, I saw a purple Papilio. He was very elusive. Time after time my net failed to ensnare him. I was in earnest, and so excited that when the beautiful creature sailed lazily over the fence, I followed.

I got a few scratches, but in my enthusiasm forgot my furbelows. When my prey crossed the creek, I lost no time, and forgetful of my beloved blue shoes, I forded the stream, and on all fours, climbed the high bank on the other side. I cast my net, and landed like a turtle on the sand. Not till I had bottled the butterfly did I notice the ruin I had wrought in my Sunday attire.

We never had any school exercises or "last day" performances in which the children speak pieces or show off before their visiting parents, but I did not feel this omission until Alice taught a district school about ten miles north of the farm. The big boys were working in the fields in the summer, and that was the reason for employing a woman teacher. Alice "boarded around", living first a few days or a week with one family and then with another, but Father and I went after her every Friday to bring her home for the week end on the farm. I was intensely interested in Alice's school, knew the names of all of the children, and when the "last day" exercises took place, I knew by heart every piece that the children spoke.

Even though I had never spoken a piece, my time came, as many things have come to me, quite unexpectedly as well as unpreparedly. It was in a religious program which took place in the district schoolhouse. Notice had been given, and at the hour set I was at the schoolhouse, in advance of all the others.

I took a seat in the back row where in school hours only the older children sat. My head came just above the desk in front of me, and my legs swung for they were not long enough to reach the floor. The piously inclined assembled, and soon the room was filled. Although Father was a confessed atheist, he was apparently glad to have me go to prayer meetings, revivals, and church whenever I wanted to.

Almeda, wife of Big Jim the farmer, was sponsoring the prayer meetings. When she and her husband drove by our house on Sunday mornings, they often saw Father with one leg of his home-made trousers draped over his boot top as he stood leaning on the front gate.

Almeda would call out, "Good morning, Joshua. Won't you come with me to find Jesus?"

Father always replied in most irreverent and uncomplimentary language, but it never discouraged the lady from repeating the invitation Sunday after Sunday.

Almeda conducted the prayer meeting. Stepping to the front of the schoolroom and crossing her hands over her round fat belly, she called out in a loud, clear, unctuous voice, "Butha, will you lead in prayer?"

Me! This was a thrust at my father—a blow below the belt. I would show her that I was a daughter worthy of my father! She would see! I rose in my seat and with great piety, really trying to look like a saint in a picture that I had seen somewhere, clasped my hands in front of me and slowly repeated The Lord's Prayer. I experienced no stage fright or timidity—in fact, nothing could have restrained me. It was my moment to vindicate my father.

When I got home, Mother was still working in the kitchen, setting the pancakes for breakfast and winding up the weights in Grandmother's old clock. I burst in with, "What do you think—Almeda asked me to lead in prayer because she wanted to run on Father."

Mother was more than interested and asked, "What did you do?" I replied, "I did."

At this juncture, Father entered with a big chunk of wood to be deposited in the great wood stove where it would burn all night long.

As Mother opened the top of the stove to help him, she remarked, "Bertha has been at the schoolhouse attending prayer meeting, and Almeda asked her to lead in prayer."

Father almost wrecked the stove, he let go of the chunk so quickly. "And what did you do?" he asked.

"I did," I answered in no casual tone.

Father's blue eyes twinkled, and with the spirit worthy of a martyr, he gave me this unstinted praise, "That's right; make them hunt their holes! Let them know there's a God in Israel!"

I had pleased my father! I had vindicated his honor! Since then I have had degrees conferred upon me, and have been honored in special ways, but nothing has ever since given me the thrill that was brought by those homely, rugged words.

6

HAYSEED GOES TO TOWN

I DESPISED my curls that had to be wound around somebody's finger every morning, and I gave Mother no peace until I was rid of them, although their loss brought Alice to the verge of tears. Because it gave me a certain freedom, I loved my Dutch dock, held back from my face with a circle comb. Because of it I felt more able to cope with the change that confronted me when Father took me to the Rochester Academy, a graded public school one and one-half miles from Stony Creek.

In good weather it was a pleasant walk over the road that Great-grandfather and his sons had cut through, forty years before I was born. However, as Rochester was our post office and trading center, Father usually found it convenient to take me back and forth with the horse and buggy.

Not until I entered this town school was I aware of the deep gulf between countryfolk and townspeople. Suddenly, for the first time, I realized that Father's boots were greased instead of shined. His trousers did not look like those of the townsman. (Little wonder, for Mother made all of them except his Sunday pair.) His hat had seen many seasons' wear, and even when new, it had been of a different vintage from urban headgear. Our horses, in winter, had long shaggy fur, the buggy was always mud-splashed, the whip was a nicely whittled stick with a leather thong at the end, and a shawl or quilt covered our laps.

Alice sensed these earmarks more keenly than I, and struggled, with some success, to introduce yard cleaning, buggy washing, table manners, fancy cooking, and modish dressing.

Reared to the dignity, security, and freedom of life on a farm, I was shocked to hear my father spoken of as "hayseed." The word "hayseed" included the clothing, manners, speech, surroundings, and even the beautiful simplicity of his character.

It seemed to me that my position as a farmer's daughter, when compared with that of one of the town children, was to my advantage. I wore better and prettier clothes, lived in a house owned by my father and enjoyed an abundance of delicious food. My father had horses and buggies, and took us to the county fair, camp meetings, Sunday School picnics, and the circus. In spite of all this, in the eyes of townspeople we were "rubes," clodhoppers, boors, rustics.

All my studies interested me, especially arithmetic. Occasionally, as early as four in the morning, I surreptitiously lighted the kerosene lamp at my bedside to finish a problem that had baffled me the night before. If Mother discovered it, and she usually did, she would creep quietly into my room and blow out the light, whispering, "You better go back to sleep and after breakfast you will have no trouble in doing your sums." As always, she was right.

During my second year in the Academy the principal asked me to teach a class in Intellectual Arithmetic. Whether he recognized my fondness for mathematics or whether he himself was overworked and needed an assistant I never learned. I was only twelve years old, and all the members of the class were older than I, but that town-versus-country gulf was so wide that I was able to teach and discipline them.

While I was still at the Rochester school, my sister was attending the Pontiac High School where one of the big events in the school year was the Junior Exhibition, when a selected number of the Junior class read original compositions before a large audience in the big hall. I was only eleven when Alice took part in such a program. Father and Mother and I were in the audience, made up largely of proud parents, and to honor the occasion I wore my blue coat, blue hood edged with swansdown and my blue kid shoes. We drove to Pontiac early enough for Mother to do some shopping and to complete my costume, she bought my first pair of kid gloves. They were white and tickled my vanity to the extent that Alice received little of my attention, for I spent the whole evening quirking my fingers and spreading them out on my blue coat.

After the exercises, on the way to Alice's boarding house where Father had left the horses, I slipped on the icy walk and fell prone on my face. Ever mindful of my beautiful new gloves, I held my hands well above the sidewalk, and in consequence was unable to get up. A gentleman passing by saw my predicament, and thinking I must be badly hurt, stooped down and lifted me bodily from the wet walk. Everyone was greatly concerned—could I stand? Could I walk? Was I in pain?

"Oh, I'm all hunky-dory," I assured them and skipped cheerfully to the wagon.

Riding home on the back seat, Alice said to me, "Why couldn't you get up? Why did that man have to pick you up like a baby if you were not hurt at all?"

Such a question amazed me and I explained how I could not get up without spoiling my new gloves. Father got a big laugh out of my presence of mind, but Alice, instead of admiring me, as I expected her to, was disgusted.

After three years in the Rochester school I was sent to Pontiac High School and entered the sophomore year. This change in schools necessitated my living in a boarding house during the five-day school week. Father came for me with the horse and buggy every Friday as soon as school closed, and brought me back on Monday in time for an eight-o'clock recitation.

For six years, three for Alice then three for me, Father put everything aside and, in all kinds of weather, made the round trip to Pontiac twice every week.

On cold, snowy winter mornings, after eating a breakfast that

Mother had prepared in time for us to leave around five o'clock, we were packed into the bobsleigh, that had been filled with sweet-smelling straw. With hot bricks that Mother had heated in the oven, and quilts and buffalo robes around us, we were ready to start. I was well protected with a woolen hood, and a long nubia wound around my head and over my face.

No matter what the weather was we were never late for school. When the scholars who lived in town came straggling into class one-half hour late, the teacher would look scornfully at them, and pointing at me, would say, "Look at Bertha Van Hoosen. She has ridden twelve miles, but she got here on time." Needless to say, this remark did not increase my popularity with my fellow students.

The boarding house in which I was placed was kept by an elderly woman and her brother who had left their farm for an easier life in town. During my first year I roomed with the daughter of a farmer living near Stony Creek, and two boys, farmers' sons, occupied a room next to ours. The rural atmosphere in this house prevented even a touch of homesickness.

Before we had begun to get acquainted with the boys, we caught sight through their half-open door of a big bag of delicious snow apples that one of them had brought from the country. With customary country freedom, we helped ourselves to the fruit whenever the boys were out of their room. We had not taken many when, one afternoon, we were horrified to find a chamber pot filled with apples placed on the table in our room. My roommate declared that she would never speak to them again, but desiring to outwit them, we did quite the opposite— invited them to play cards with us that evening.

We left the disgraceful chamber pot in the center of the table, but covered and concealed it with a thick mat of beautiful autumn foliage. The rosy fruit on the background of crimson and yellow maple leaves was really atractive, and like tempting Eves, we spent the evening urging the boys to eat an apple, and giggling and blushing over their embarrassed refusal. After this episode we became life-long friends.

This social function, however, was not repeated, for every evening was spent studying. I could have graduated when I was fifteen, but since I could not enter the University of Michigan until I was sixteen, I continued an extra year in high school. I took French and German, in addition to Greek and Latin, and thus obtained college credit for two extra languages.

I did well enough in all my studies, but the sole satisfaction that I derived from good marks was in reporting them to Father as we jogged along, over the dirt roads on Friday afternoons. One week, when we had a particularly dreaded examination in geometry, Father asked me, "Did you pass?"

I bristled, "I got 99.8!"

"Why didn't you get 100?"

"No one in the class did. I was the highest one."

"That's right! Make them hunt their holes. Let them know there's a God in Israel." Father began whistling, slapped the horse's back with the reins, and it seemed to me I could never be any happier.

Alice was in college all during the years I spent in high school, but we came back to the farm for our vacations. At home we read together, played games or helped Mother. I never played any games in school or with my schoolmates, but I was quite familiar with dominoes and croquet because I could play these games alone and enjoy them quite as much as with a companion. However, I lost my zeal for croquet at an afternoon party at the home of one of Alice's aristocratic town friends. Proud of the invitation, I wore a blue dress trimmed with double plaitings that were fringed on both edges, and cream-colored stockings with conspicuous clocks of blue grapes that Alice had embroidered with an eye to my costume's color scheme.

I was almost a professional in croquet and if I had the good fortune to play first in a game, I often made every wicket before my opponent had a chance to begin. Stimulated by the thought that Alice would be proud of me, I played a winning game, but frequently had to stop and pull up my stockings.

When Alice could stand it no longer, she sidled up to me as

I was poised for a stroke and whispered in my ear, "What is the matter with your stockings?"

In surprise I answered, "Nothing. I just forgot my 'lastics."

My ardor vanished before her embarrassment, and no success in the game could restore it.

It was not, however, surprising that I forgot the garters, for I had never worn shoes in the summer until I was sixteen years of age, except on such grand occasions as a grown-up party away from home.

My graduation from high school would have been a bright spot in my adolescence if it had not been preceded by a crushing breakdown in my moral standards.

No one in the family ever lied. To Mother, honesty was a Bible injunction. To Father, honesty was a manifestation of common sense and good business principles. To Alice, honesty was evidence of good breeding and culture. Up to my senior year in high school I had never been tempted to lie. Then suddenly, in a moment of false security, sin claimed me.

During my last two years in Pontiac I roomed with a young woman, Alida Deland, who was several years older than I and a person of fine character and mature judgment. At that time she was engaged to Samuel W. Smith, whom she later married. Her husband, in time, was elected senator from Michigan, term after term. Sammie gratified Father's Republican pride.

Although Sammie and Alida were very Victorian in their courting, they must have stimulated my dormant social appetite to some extent. It was through them, although they were not aware of it, that for the first time I broke the commandment, "Thou shalt not bear false witness."

One evening Mr. Smith came to call on Alida, as he often did, and suggested going to Detroit to see Booth in "Hamlet." Mr. Smith had a lawyer friend who, he said, would like to take me. We could go into Detroit on the evening train, and return on the midnight.

I had never ridden on a train, never been to a theater, and had never had an escort. It was a big order for one evening.

They planned to go Friday night. Father would come for me Friday afternoon as usual, to take me home. I could get his permission when he came and go home Saturday, instead of Friday. I had never met Mr. Smith's friend, but had heard Father speak of him as a "squirt." I was so positive that Father would not approve of my going with him that when I asked his permission, I did not mention my escort's name, but said that Alida and Smith wanted me to go with them.

Father thought it over. "My, I know what it means to you—but it seems to me too much for Mr. Smith to do."

"Well," I said, "Smith and Alida want me to go."

After a thoughtful look at me he nodded. "All right, we will come after you tomorrow morning."

He drove away, and at that moment my punishment began. I had been taught that a lie was any statement that conveyed a false impression. That I had not made a statement that was, per se, false did not mean to me that I had not lied to my father.

Alida was very happy that I was going to go, but I was suffering even before we left for the train. Alida and I sat opposite the two men, and I felt myself growing more and more serious and sad. I couldn't bear to look at the man whom I now considered responsible for all my unhappiness.

Upon reaching Detroit we went to a hotel to have dinner and brush up for the evening. I had no appetite, and would have been glad to stay alone in the room at the hotel.

The theater was so enormous that I felt lost in it, but only a moment, for just three seats ahead of us I spied the village doctor who had been called to officiate at the time of my birth. Now there was no escape. I could almost hear Dr. Wilson saying to Father, "Hello, there! So you are going to have a new son-in-law soon! I saw Bertha at the theater with Mr. Trip."

My misery was so great that I held my program in front of my face most of the time. I could not enjoy or even hear the words of the great actor. When at the end of the play most of the actors lay dead, I envied them.

We rode back to Pontiac, facing the men, and when we walked

47

from the train to the boarding house, I refused to take my escort's arm and replied to his solicitous questions apathetically. When we reached the gate, I rushed through, without even saying good night to my "betrayer."

Long before old Beck and the buggy drew up, I was watching and waiting for Father. Instead of Father I found Aunt Julia who was staying a few months with us, as she often did.

As soon as we were well on our way, Aunt Julia asked me, "Did you have a grand time?"

"No," I confessed. "I had a bad time. I lied to Father. I went with Mr. Trip, and Alida went with Mr. Smith."

Aunt Julia did not seem to think things were so desperate, but I was inconsolable.

Seeing dinner on the table when we arrived, I took off my hat and sat down. Father served me in the quantities I liked, but by this time I was almost exploding. Looking at, but not seeing my plate, I said, "Father, I lied to you. I went with Mr. Trip, and Alida went with Mr. Smith."

Silence ensued. I glanced up and saw tears rolling down Father's ruddy cheeks. "I'm sorry," was all he said.

I left the table and went to the spare bedroom where I threw myself on the bed and gave way to uncontrollable grief. After a time Mother came and sympathized with me. "You have had a hard lesson, but it may be the best thing that ever has happened to you." She, as usual, convinced me that "Whatever is, is right" and I again appeared in public, a humble convert to the honesty-is-the-best-policy way of life.

As long as Father was alive, everyone in the family had an individual pocketbook. Father had *the* pocketbook. Mother had another replenished with butter and egg sales. Alice's pocketbook was filled with money given her by Father and Mother. The contents of my pocketbook depended upon my success in hunting eggs.

Fall after fall when the time came for Alice to return to college, I had experienced a tension in the atmosphere. It was the time when roosters began to crow, and I never have been able to disassociate the efforts of the young cock from a feeling of worry about money and a fear of finding Mother behind some door, crying because her daughter was going away.

Mother and Alice would go into a huddle, and then Mother would stage the assault on Father. He would produce his wallet and in rapt silence count out the money Alice was to take. Mother and Alice talked over the money question with great frankness, but there seemed to be some barrier between them and Father when it came to money matters, though we all knew that our going to college was the realization of my father's dream.

I never knew the time when it was not a foregone conclusion that I was to go to college. I seemed to have been born with that end in view, congenitally catalogued for college. I determined that when it came my turn, I would institute a new regime. I told Mother I was going to talk the money question over with Father. She seemed surprised, and a little perturbed.

After dinner Father always lingered at the table and allowed the cat to walk over his shoulders and make furtive passes at his plate until he finally gave her a few bits to eat. I took this opportunity to present my financial program. "Father," I said, "I have figured it all out, and it will cost me three hundred dollars for the year in college. I would like to have that amount, and spend it as I need it."

Father said, "You couldn't get through on that amount," but I replied, "I will! And what's more, I'll send you an expense account every time I need more money."

Father looked at me. "Now, Bertha," he said, "I have plenty of money for you to live in a comfortable way in Ann Arbor, but—I have not one cent for you to futter away. Your mother and I work hard, but we want you to have everything you need If you want to try the way you say, it is all right with me."

That ended Mother's function as a money go-between. Father always sent me money whenever I needed any and the plan was happy for everybody. However, the desirability of a common family purse began to shape itself in my mind at this time and continued to grow after this experience.

TURN THE OTHER CHEEK....

MY SISTER and I were diametrically opposite in looks, disposition, tastes and physique. She was a brunette and I had red hair like my father. She was mercurial, alert and self-conscious; I was more phlegmatic and self-absorbed. But one thing we had in common was an admiration and deep love for each other. Mother did much to crystallize this by never allowing us to quarrel.

When I was about six and Alice fourteen, we were in the cellar where we did the weekly or semi-weekly churning. We had an old dash churn and I was pushing the dasher from side to side instead of lifting it up and pushing it down. Alice, in a kindly tone, asked me to stop pushing the dasher that way.

For a few times I lifted it, but as it became heavy, I began again to push it from side to side. Alice lost her temper and gave me a smart slap on my ear. She had never done anything like that before. I considered the matter and decided that if I let this pass she might repeat her action at some other time, so I made up my mind to hit back. I quickly raised my arm and gave her as near a "Joe Louis" return as I was able. It surprised her as much as it hurt her. Then we both began to cry.

We made up in a hurry and nothing like it ever happened again. Alice thought she was the more excusable because she did it impetuously and I did it deliberately. I felt I was less culpable because I was forced to it in self-defense.

7

INVITATION TO MEDICINE

IN 1880, I entered the Literary Department of the University of Michigan with a year's credit in French and German. My first year in college gave me a peep into a world, the value of which I had never before been able to fathom or understand.

My long heavy titian hair wound about my head like a cap, my high coloring and little apron accentuated my youth. The apron was Alice's idea, and every day I wore a fresh one of white muslin with narrow lace trimming and ties in the back. None of the other girls wore aprons or arranged their hair in coronet braids, but if my appearance pleased Alice, that was all that was necessary.

Undoubtedly my costume caught the fancy of Charles Mills Gailey, teacher of Latin, and glamour man of the faculty.

In the early spring, at the close of the lesson on the love poems of Catullus, Professor Gailey asked me, along with some of the other students, to remain after class. I was greatly perturbed, and became more so when he interviewed student after student and left me waiting.

Finally I was alone with this fascinating Irishman, who, with a heart-robbing smile said, "I am sorry to have kept you waiting. I wanted only to ask you if you received gentlemen callers."

Greatly relieved, I blurted out, "I never did, but I would."

"May I come tonight?"

I consented and this was the beginning of many unforgettable evenings together. We were walking in the twilight one evening when he apparently accidentally placed his hand over mine. I wriggled it away, but a new and strange feeling flooded me. It was something of which I had never before been sensible.

When we parted one night, he took both my hands in his. At this juncture, I gave a vocal exposition of my mental state. "I believe you are a bad man." He dropped my hands, turned and left. The next evening he returned to ask why I had said such a dreadful thing.

"I am here alone," I explained, "without my parents who expect me to take care of myself. You are my teacher, and I expect you to treat me as my parents would wish me to be treated. If you had been one of my classmates, I should have slapped you."

I did not tell him that I had often heard Father say in speaking of delinquent girls, "My girls can choose their own companions and marry anyone they want to, but if they get blistered, they will have to sit on the blisters, not I."

In all my pre-college experience I had never heard of a woman physician. My freshman curiosity was therefore whetted when I learned that the two young ladies who were living in a boarding-house across the street from the sorority house were studying medicine.

They were Vassar products. One of them, Mary McLean, a tall, pale, mettlesome young woman, but a cultured Southern lady withal, was religious to a degree that approached bigotry; the other, Harriet Barringer, was refined and dignified, but more than that, an eye-catcher in a college town. She wore for everyday a long ermine cape and a hat made of peacock feathers. Often, when asked why I selected medicine as a career, I have been tempted to reply, "It was a peacock hat and ermine coat that first attracted me to the medical profession."

The fact that these girls were "hen-medics" did not deter me, as it did my sorority sisters, from making their acquaintance at once. Yet it was only after long and cautious consideration where curiosity was the scale-tipping factor, that the die was cast to call on them. Their enthusiasm for their work fired my imagination.

My friendship with Mary McLean and Harriet Barringer, and the attentions of my Latin teacher, Professor Charles Gailey, did much towards my coming of age. When I returned to the farm at the end of my freshman year in the literary department, Alice said mournfully, "You left a little girl and come back a woman."

In my sophomore year I deliberately elected a social career for my major subject. In order to avoid the repetition of a near-flunk in history my freshman year, I took as few hours as the authorities allowed, choosing only courses known as "snaps."

For my social career I deemed it necessary to join a tennis club, a whist club made up of young faculty members, and a dancing class. I attended one or two dances every week, went to all kinds of entertainments, and when there was nothing else going on, played poker with my roommate and a bunch of college boys who were always ready and waiting to join us.

My dancing must have been a trial to my partners until I learned to allow them to hug me tight enough to propel me around as the turtle carries its shell, my feet only now and then touching the floor. The necessary sense of keeping time to the music I never acquired.

My skating was even worse—possibly the fault of my ankles that seemed to have a ball-bearing action. Whenever I tried to stand or slide, I would find myself sitting, jack-knifing, lying flat, or kneeling on the ice, unable to move until someone came to the rescue. However, when it came to coasting down the steep Ann Arbor hills, I could guide the sled whether I was standing, sitting spoon-fashion, or lying "belly-gut", and walking back up hill brought into play all of the muscles I had developed in my childhood playground.

I was first choice for partner at whist, and poker fascinated me, although we never played for money. When it came to money, Hetty Green, New York City's woman millionaire, was my financial guide. I paid two dollars and fifty cents for twenty-one meals and the same amount per week for my room. This left one hundred dollars for all my other expenses during the college year; sufficient, providing "not one cent was futtered away."

I worked so hard on my social career that at the end of my sophomore year I had passed through the stages of amateur and professional, and was ready for retirement. Since then no post-graduate or refresher course has ever tempted me.

Before this time I had never considered what I would do with my life, but now, although there were few vocations open to women and fewer suitable for a college-educated woman, I turned my attention to the subject with positive ferocity.

I did not seek, nor could I have got help from any of my family. They only laughed when, cross-legged like a Grand Lama in front of his prayer wheel, I took a seat on Mother's haircloth sofa, with my face towards its round black back, and announced, "I am going to sit here till my mind is made up about what I am going to do the rest of my life."

My recently acquired maturity urged that my career be chosen at once, but three days elapsed before I abandoned my haircloth seat, convinced that medicine offered women more than any other occupation.

One by one I marshaled the advantages and the disadvantages of a medical career and charted them in their respective columns. Marriage had to be seriously considered, for few women, unless they have spiritual ambitions, wish voluntarily to deprive themselves of matrimonial opportunities. In a medical career marrying, bearing children, and managing a home is not incompatible with interval practice or a complete resumption of activity at any time or in any place after an interruption.

Under any circumstances I wished marriage to play the same part in my life that it does in the life of a man, and before marriage to be prepared for a possible incompetency on the part of my husband, as well as for widowhood. Medicine answered this challenge.

Nor was I willing, after devoting years to preparation for my life work, at the climax of my efficiency to be retired because of age. As a physician this could never happen, for I could continue in practice as long as patients had confidence in me, and my health permitted.

I wanted to be my own boss—to say as Father often did, "I can speak my mind on any subject, and the corn will continue to ripen and the cows to give down their milk. I am a free man." The physician deals with all ages and with individuals of superior, as well as equal attainments. In medicine I would find use for every aptitude, and a variety of work offered through specializations. I recognized the attractiveness of the material necessities mandatory in the practice of medicine: a horse and buggy (now an automobile), an office, a home, and personal servants.

It would be a pleasant sensation to feel that I was one of the "indispensable" citizens in the community. Many physicians hold such positions of dignity.

Social status would be accorded me as a member of a learned profession, and for the same reason memberships in various medical and lay societies would promote friendships and pleasant acquaintances.

At the head of the column, however, I placed the opportunity for growth and advancement in an ever-expanding science—constant reading and studying to keep abreast with medical progress.

Perhaps, after all, in my choice of a medical career, unconsciously I was responding to a call of the woman in me—woman, preserver of the race—to mitigate suffering and save life.

Of one thing I am certain. It was not the urge for money that influenced my choice, even though my financial need was great.

I had also considered the disadvantages, the greatest of which was the power of medical practice to possess the entire time and interest of its followers. Loss of sleep, irregular meals, exposure to weather, and contact with disease are characters that spell life—life in all its fullness, and I was not afraid of life.

The Bible says, "Ye must be born again." After making my choice of a medical career, as far as the conduct of my life was concerned, I suffered a rebirth.

During my junior year I accepted no social invitations and elected as much work as was allowed without special permission. After consultation with my friends in the medical department, I selected subjects that I thought might be helpful in my study of medicine: qualitative and quantitative inorganic chemistry, organic chemistry, toxicology, assaying of ores, hygiene and sanitation, and a course in histology.

Medical students at the present time are required to take two or three years of premedic study before entering medical school and unconsciously, I created for myself the analogue of today's entrance requirements. When I listen to the difficulties that medical students encounter in the study of chemistry, I wonder if my selection of so many courses in that science was not wise and fortunate. "Snaps" no longer interested me. I worked with all my might and main and was conspicuous, not for burning the traditional midnight oil, but for flirting with Aurora. I rose quite regularly at three or four o'clock every morning to study, and this country habit has never left me. My favorite hour for operating is seven or seven-thirty in the morning when everything is spotless, everyone fresh, and no one, except the person attending to her business, is about.

The premedic courses that I had elected bristled with interest, and became a daily stimulus for the career that had become my obsession. I never mentioned my ambitions to any of the college girls, but my family knew that I thought only in terms of medicine. Mother, in her powerful passiveness, was opposed to my studying medicine; and Father, feeling that he must not act contrary to her wishes, said, "Your mother cries whenever your studying medicine is mentioned, and I cannot furnish money for you to do something that hurts her so much. Why not teach school, or better still, come home and stay with us."

Utterly disregarding these generous suggestions, I replied with verve, "I don't want your money—I can earn it."

"All right. You earn the money and spend it in any way you want to," he acquiesced.

Having entered college with advanced credit in French and German, I completed requirements for my A.B. degree at the end of the first semester of my senior year. In the hope that I might receive credit for a year in medicine before taking my degree in June, I entered the medical department at once.

Just before entering medical school, I attended one of the classes to find out how it would feel to be a medical student. The classroom was nearly full when one of the women students, wearing a hat with red roses, entered. The boys made a clucking sound, and some threw paper wads and kisses. I recalled my district-school days when I did not dare to wear a new coat lest I be called "stuck-up." I outwitted those country children by maltreating the coat till it looked old, and now I must elude these men students.

Without delay I bought enough black material (black always was, and is still unbecoming to me) for a dress, and made it as simple and plain as a nun's habit, unconsciously adding to its artlessness by wearing a black plush bonnet guiltless of trimming, and tied with black strings under my chin.

Not relying too much on this costume for my protection, I exercised care never to raise my eyes from the ground going to and from class, and when in class I directed my attention to the professor.

I flattered myself that I typified a formal and reserved person, such as my mother appeared to be and really was. However, in retrospect, I am positive that I looked naive and quaint—the opposite of what I was striving to attain.

I maneuvered my entrance into medicine with such secrecy that it was six weeks before any of my friends found it out. The cat was out of the bag when I accidentally dropped one of my medical text books on the floor of the sorority house, and a curious sorority sister spelled slowly "M-A-T-E-R-I-A M-E-D-I-C-A," and gasped, "Are you studying medicine?"

Everybody was excited and seemed to regard me with special

interest and awed admiration. Yet, no one ruffled my feathers by calling "Hen medic!"

Having received my A.B. degree in June, 1884, I arranged to continue my medical studies in the fall, and to pay my expenses by waiting on table for my board and room. With summer vacation before me, my need for money translated the time into an opportunity for work instead of play. With the farm as my center for operating, I sold scales to the farmers' wives in the neighborhood, but many wanted to enjoy a visit with me and treated me so like the prodigal son that I could not talk business. I gave up peddling scales and turned to picking berries, for two cents a quart.

In August Dr. McLean wrote, "There is an opening in the Mary Institute here in St. Louis, to teach calisthenics and physiology." This school was then a popular high-grade grammar and high school, now preparatory for the Washington University.

Dr. Mary McLean, who had inspired me to study medicine, had just started to practice in St. Louis and knew that I was planning to finance my way through medical school. As I had never been even inside a gymnasium, and knew nothing at all about calisthenics, I wrote her regretting that I was not competent to take the position.

Her reply astounded me. "I have secured the position for you. Don't worry about the calisthenics. Come to St. Louis a couple of weeks before school opens, and take some instructions."

Alice argued, "Why don't you try teaching? After all, you might like it; anyway it will be a more pleasant way to earn money than waiting on table while going to school, or doing all the menial jobs you have done this summer. Father and Mother would love to have you teach school."

In all my problems Alice is always the precipitating drop that clears the solution.

Early in September, Dr. McLean met me in St. Louis and took me to her front-and-back-parlor office which served also as living room and bedroom. Dr. McLean occupied the bed, while I slept on a couch—but not alone, for I was given a warm and bloodthirsty welcome by the inhabitants of that berth. There were no bugs in Mother's beds or in any that I occupied in Ann Arbor. This was my first encounter, and as I gazed ruefully at my blood-bespattered gown, Dr. McLean in her quick, decisive manner announced, "We will move at once."

Dr. McLean's religious scruples that permitted no reading on Sunday, except the Bible, did not prevent me from buying the Sunday paper and marking about forty places where we might find suitable accommodations. All day Monday was spent in a search that proved utterly hopeless. The rooming house owners were unanimous on two points: no woman doctor, and no sign, even if the sign were no bigger than a postage stamp.

We attempted a solution of the problem by looking at furnished or unfurnished houses, but this was as baffling as finding a room. No real estate firm would rent Dr. McLean a house unless she signed a contract never to put a sign on it, or even a doorplate with Dr. or M.D. attached to her name. The reason they gave was the fear that it would place such a stigma on the house that they could never rent it again.

At our wits' end, we advertised for rooms, and to our surprise and delight, found a front-and-back parlor heated by a grate in each room, in a house on Olive Street, not far from the Mary Institute where I was going to teach. A few weeks after we moved in we learned that we were living in a neighborhood appropriately called "Scab Row," and I am sure that that was the explanation of our success in solving our housing problem.

Actually, our embarrassment over this epithet was less distressing than the discovery that the landlady's small children used the front entrance of the house as a toilet. Yet no patient was ever shocked by such a nuisance. No patients ever came. After Dr. McLean had had an office in St. Louis for more than a year, she was still waiting for her first patient.

In my initiation into medicine, Dr. McLean opened my eyes to the prejudice, the discrimination, the lack of confidence and paucity of opportunities that had to be reckoned with before success could be secured.

The day after my arrival Dr. McLean invited me to a clinic at the City Hospital. Seated in the big amphitheater, the pit of which was filled with patients in wheel chairs, I was enjoying watching the interns do the surgical dressings until I saw a probe go boring down deep into a wound—the whole room began to whirl around and go into a tail spin.

In a faraway voice I heard Dr. McLean say, "We will go now."

I followed her, my heels clicking against the floor, for I could hardly lift them. We finally reached a bed, where, after lying down a very few minutes, I recovered.

Her remark, "Traveling has made you a little wobbly; it will not happen again," did not remove my swoon complex, for when we went to the Mullanphy Hospital, my humiliating experience was repeated, although I had had a week to recuperate.

The room in which this gynecological clinic was held was partitioned to accommodate patients on one side and students on the other. The partition was broken in the center by a curtain, and through this space an examining table could be pushed.

Dr. McLean explained the technique: "The nurse arranges the patient on the table, and after covering her with a sheet, pushes it through the opening to the student side, the curtain falling down upon the patient. This leaves the patient's head and torso on the patient side and her pelvis convenient for the students to examine."

Our seats were in the front row—I heard the patient climb upon the table—the curtain swayed—the covered legs and exposed sexual organs of the patient came into view—my eyes blurred, and I felt the floor sinking.

Doctor grasped my hand. "Come," she pressed.

With difficulty I followed her, dragging my feet like a paralytic's.

I heard her indulgent, "Everything is so new here, I think it is too much for you to attend clinics and do the school work."

Incredulous, I said nothing.

When, on the following Saturday, Dr. McLean said, "You had better stay at home and rest," I announced, "I am not only going, but I am going to stay till I faint, and when I come to, I am going to remain, no matter how many times I faint."

We took front seats as usual, and sure enough, as soon as the curtain moved, and the table came nosing its way into the student side of the partition, I became ghastly faint.

Dr. McLean reached for my hand. "Come!" she insisted.

I shook my head.

"Come!" she repeated.

I shook my head until the hairpins loosened and my hair, like Lady Godiva's, threatened to cover my shame.

She urged, "Do come."

I turned towards her, and said doggedly, "No!" and at this word all my faintness vanished, never to return at any time.

Dr. McLean was so proud and hopeful that she would not ask for money till it was absolutely necessary—after she had used up all the money her father had sent and then all my monthly salary.

Her father, a retired physician residing in a small town near St. Louis, was anxious to see his daughter established in a successful practice and sent her a check whenever she needed money.

One Saturday morning, when Dr. McLean was expecting money, the combined exchecquer was down to carfare to the post office, but no letter came either in the morning or afternoon. We had been having our meals sent in, but when Dr. McLean asked, "Can we pay on Monday?" the reply was, "No money, no meals."

Sunday morning, quite sure that the letter and check would be at the post office, the doctor spent our last dime for carfare, but returned empty-handed.

Dr. McLean was on delicately intimate terms with God, asking his advice about the weather and even social obligations—"Dear God, shall I wear my raincoat this morning?" or "Heavenly Father, what do you think about my asking the judge and his family to dinner next Sunday?"

In later years when she had acquired a large practice and was one of the leading surgeons in St. Louis, it was her custom to open the abdomen with a prayer; like the opening of a political convention where prayer is offered for the opposing party.

I was not surprised, therefore, when she suggested that we devote the day to prayer and the study of the Bible, disregarding the cries of every tissue in the body for nourishment. However, the advantage of my physical make-up, stimulated by calisthenics, over my spiritual state was so great that everything I read suggested food, and the only prayer I could force from my lips was "Give us this day our daily bread." With the advent of Monday came the check, and the starvelings were able to substitute for one meal in three days, three meals in one.

I was such a congenital Pollyanna that a physiological bellyache was only a new and interesting sensation, and Dr. McLean was such a religious zealot that a little haircloth only incited her longing for holiness. Nevertheless, one day when the doctor returned from her daily walk, she found me in tears. Hoping that I might pass off one or two courses when I returned to medical school, I had chosen anatomy as one of the most important freshman courses, and had set out to memorize it. After reading a page, I tried to recall what I had read, but my mind was a blank. I tried to remember one-half of a page—nothing registered. Then I tried one paragraph—Father had suspected the truth, when I was a little girl and he feared I was a moron. My inferiority complex took possession of me and was tearing my medical career into shreds when Dr. McLean rescued me by explaining that anatomy was a subject that could not be memorized, but had to be learned in the dissecting room, sitting by the side of a cadaver.

At the end of her first year of waiting, Dr. McLean was appointed resident physician to the Female Hospital. This was a part of the St. Louis City Hospital, devoted to the care of veneral diseases in women. It was a turning point in her life, for although internships were neither required nor even customary for medical students, they were as important a part of medical education then, as they are now.

She approached her hospital service seriously and devoted night and day to her patients. Still, she was very lonely, and I went twice a week to visit her. To reach the Female Hospital, I rode to the end of the streetcar line, walked miles across the park to the hospital, saving the twenty-five cent bus fare, and arrived just in time for supper. Afterwards, we walked up and down stairs into ward after ward until nine o'clock. By this time almost walking in my sleep, I undressed and went to bed; but the doctor stayed up for hours, writing histories and reading about puzzling cases. We shared her single hospital bed, and after she had joined me, I would be rudely wakened to find her, in her sleep, percussing my lungs, or taking my pulse.

Dr. McLean was the first woman to serve in any official capacity in any hospital in St. Louis. Her record was so exceptionally high and so unusual that few men in the profession did not know of her accomplishments as a skillful operator and an exhaustive diagnostician. In fact, she was better known after that year's service in the Female Hospital than many physicians after practicing for a lifetime. When she again began to practice in St. Louis, she had the unique experience of being the fad. Society women, church women, and the families of men physicians flocked to her office, which she had set up in her comfortabe home.

I had still three months to teach when she left me to begin her residency, but feeling responsible for me, she found a very pleasant, high-grade boarding house where I stayed till school closed.

As much as I had enjoyed teaching, when Dr. Purnell, the principal, said, "Will you teach another year? We will, of course, increase your salary," I answered, "No, I intend to study medicine, and have too little confidence in myself not to keep my eye on the goal."

He put his arm around me and confided, "I once wanted to be a lawyer, but I kept on teaching because I had a good job: then I married and had a family—well, I am still teaching. You are a wise little girl. Keep to your singleness of purpose."

THE HIPPOCRATIC OATH

I SWEAR by Apollo the physician, and Aesculapius, and Hygeia, and Panacea, and all the gods and goddesses, that, according to my ability and judgment, I will keep this Oath and this stipulation—to reckon him who taught me this art equally dear to me as my parents, to share my substance with him, and relieve his necessities if required; to look upon his offspring in the same footing as my own brothers, and teach them this art, if they shall wish to learn it, without fee or stipulation, and that by precept, lecture and every other mode of instruction, I will impart a knowledge of the art to my own sons, and those of my teachers, and to disciples bound by a stipulation and oath according to the law of medicine, but to none others. I will follow that system of regimen which, according to my ability and judgment, I consider for the benefit of my patients, and abstain from whatever is deleterious and mischievous. I will give no deadly medicine to anyone if asked, nor suggest any such counsel; and in like manner I will not give to a woman a pessary to produce abortion; with purity and holiness I will pass my life and practice my art. I will not cut persons laboring under the stone, but will leave this to be done by men who are practitioners of this work. Into whatever houses I enter, I will go into them for the benefit of the sick, and will abstain from every voluntary act of mischief and corruption; and, further, from the seduction of females or males, of freemen and slaves. Whatever, in connection with my professional practice or not in connection with it, I see and hear in the life of men which ought not to be spoken of abroad, I will not divulge, as reckoning that all such should be kept secret. While I continue to keep this Oath unviolated, may it be granted to me to enjoy life and the practice of the art, respected by all men, in all times! But should I trespass and violate this Oath, may the reverse be my lot!

8

"I SWEAR BY APOLLO...."

IN THE FALL of 1885 I presented my credentials to the University of Michigan Medical School. Nevertheless, before I could be given a year's credit, I was required to conform to the rule of the University and take an oral examination in all freshman courses in the presence of the assembled heads of departments. I took the vacant chair at the long faculty table. Each professor asked as many questions as he wished, and then and there gave his report.

Since I had studied materia medica for only two months, I expected to be either conditioned or not passed, but instead, Dr. Vaughn, acting for the absent professor, spoke up, "I will pass Miss Van Hoosen without any examination whatever.

In chemistry, where I was more than prepared and expected to shine, I was told, "I will pass Miss Van Hoosen, but will require her to listen to the freshman lectures in chemistry."

Without exception the teachers and the men students in the medical school were fair and friendly to the women. The anathemas against "hen medics" came from the students in the literary department, both men and women.

Not until I entered the medical school did I encounter real teachers, and then only two, Dr. Corydon L. Ford and Dr. Victor C. Vaughn. It was Dr. Vaughn, Dean of the University of

Michigan Medical School, who taught me, though belatedly, that I did not know my lesson unless I knew everything remotely related to it as well as everything directly connected with it.

Dr. Ford, head and professor of Anatomy, was a master teacher, and the student who could not learn from him must have been both blind and deaf. Lame, his rugged bearded face lined with the dignity and responsibilities of his profession, he was an inspiring picture as he delivered an anatomy lecture to those unschooled medical students, poorly prepared to begin the scientific study of medicine. A high school diploma was the only entrance requirement, and many students were working for their board and room.

Dr. Ford would enter the lecture amphitheater, lay aside his cane, uncover the cadaver and then, pointing to the groin, would say, "Inguinal region, gentlemen, inguinal region. We will study today the inguinal region. My hand is lying on the inguinal region, gentlemen. Inguinal region. This region is covered with integument. I lift the integument and show the fascia beneath . . . femoral artery, gentlemen. Finger pointing to femoral artery. Pencil tapping femoral artery. Femoral artery, gentlemen . . . Femoral vein, gentlemen. Finger pointing to femoral vein. Pencil tapping femoral vein. Femoral vein, gentlemen. . . ."

In this repetitious manner, he visually and didactically demonstrated every structure in the cadavar. Study was unnecessary after listening to Dr. Ford's lecture, for he branded it into the brain and retina of the dullest dolt. Oliver Wendell Holmes paid him this tribute, "It is worth a trip to Europe and back again, to hear an anatomy lecture by Corydon L. Ford."

During the passing years the knowledge of medicine, surgery, pediatrics, obstetrics, gynecology, physiology and materia medica that I acquired in medical school has slowly, bit by bit, become obsolete. Meanwhile in the never-closing school of medical practice, I have studied anesthesia, metabolism, serology, cardiography, roentgenology, endocrinology, aseptic surgery, physiotherapy, preventive medicine—a list with no end in sight.

While discoveries are being made in many fields and changes have taken place in other branches of medicine, anatomy remains the same, yesterday, today, and forever.

Although the University of Michigan gave me a magnificent anatomical foundation for surgery, the surgical instruction that they gave at that time is now archaic; the inspiration only has continued unchanged throughout the years.

The specialty of surgery has always been regarded with favor and admiration. Many of the surgeons at the time I graduated had received their training in the Civil War, and among them was Dr. Donald McLean, my Professor of Surgery. He was a tall, handsome, blond Scotchman with a ruddy complexion and a manner suggestive of great folks. He told us there was really nothing in the germ theory, that it was fantastic and would be short-lived. Dr. Sullivan, his assistant, was laughed at heartily when Dr. McLean discovered him operating under a carbolic spray.

If he had accepted the germ theory, it would certainly have wrecked his dramatic technique. Although it is almost three score years since I sat, all eyes and ears, in his clinic, I have never since seen any surgery as dashing. Close-shaven, with linen spotless and clothes freshly pressed, he entered the operating room, laid aside his coat, and rolled back his shirt sleeves on which there was never the slightest tinge of soil—even on the inside of the cuffs. Next, he slipped on a rubber apron that had the appearance of being new, so fresh and clean it was. A rubber sheet with a slit to expose the abdomen, was placed over the patient's body.

Dr. McLean meticulously selected the bistowry—it, too, seemed new, so bright and shiny was the steel!

For a fraction of a second only he poised the blade above the abdomen; then, swift as a bird of prey, the sharp lancet shot through all the layers of the abdomen, skin, fascia, muscle, and peritoneum, into the distended cystic tumor. Dropping the knife, his hand followed through the incision, down deeply enough to grasp the very bottom of the cyst and turn it wrong side out as he dragged it from the abdomen. Then he cut the pedicle of the tumor, and ligated it with white braided silk, closing the abdomen with the same suture material.

The wound healed with plenty of laudable pus, which was looked upon as a normal and desirable condition. The fact that Dr. McLean's mortality rate was not high is evidence that speed and accuracy are as important as asepsis.

The time filled with days of study passed quickly, but it did not vanish so rapidly as my money. Determined to keep studying until I had become reduced to my last penny, I applied to the Woman's Hospital in Detroit for the position of medical-student nurse during the summer vacation.

This summer service had been in operation for several years, but the hospital matron who acted as superintendent had nothing good to say of my predecessors. Naturally I had difficulty in obtaining the position, which was in a sense a probation opportunity to recoup their failures. Although I was anxious to get my college quota of obstetrical deliveries, I was fearful that my knowledge of nursing, summed up in "what every woman knows", would not be sufficient.

Ignorant, but young, country-bred, and willing, I attacked my duties with enthusiasm.

Eager to witness a childbirth, I did not have long to wait. The labor was well advanced when the call came, and disregarding the protestations of the matron and supervising nurses, I left my dinner untouched and hurried to the ward where the patient, screened from view of four others, was laboring.

She was pushing with her feet against a board (a table leaf) set up at the foot of the bed, while each hand grasped a knotted sheet that had been twisted into a rope and fastened to the bed. I took a position at the foot of the bed where I could have an unobstructed view of the delivery.

I congratulated myself on arriving in time. It would be over in a few minutes, I thought. However, the progress of the patient, who insisted that she could not bear down on account of the pain, did not please the doctor.

"As soon as you feel the pain, take a deep breath, close your mouth, and bear down just as you would for a movement of the bowels. There now! Take a deep breath, and press down. Oh, don't scream like that, or you will never give birth to your baby." The doctor repeated similar admonitions with each pain, but still there was no sign of the birth.

For a long time there was no change. Then the patient began voluntarily to bear down. Her facial muscles contorted, and her whole body took part in a supreme effort to expel the child.

Greatly encouraged, both doctor and nurse urged excitedly, in one breath, "Hang on to that! Don't let it go! Hold your breath!" As futile as her efforts had been before, now nothing could restrain those powerful impulses for expulsion. The patient's face grew purple. Her brow was beaded with sweat that trickled down her face. Her hands were swollen from pulling on the sheets. Her breath came in quick gasps. Her nostrils were distended and her eyes suffused. The atmosphere of the birth chamber was filled with hope and courage, for with every pain some tiny portion of the baby's head became increasingly visible.

The patient was now instructed to cease bearing down, lest harmful tears might result. With each pain the doctor called loudly, "Open your mouth! Scream! Don't bear down!" Endeavoring to prevent too rapid birth, the doctor actually pushed back the head, which like the shaven circle of the bishop's scalp, appeared and disappeared until the birth could no longer be delayed. Then, suddenly, the head, followed quickly by the body, lay in a limp mass between the mother's legs.

A sharp cry was heard. The baby's arms and legs struck out aimlessly, and all wet and covered with white flecks, it lay a helpless victor in the race with life and death.

Here, as student nurse in the Woman's Hospital, my physical, mental and emotional systems were kept at such a high pitch of activity that it became impossible for me to relax or rest. Night after night, as soon as I fell asleep, I jumped out of my bed and started to remake it. At this point I wakened, but again and again, when I lost consciousness, I repeated the performance. I outmaneuvered this emotional manifestation by sleeping on the bare mattress devoid of all bed clothing. Towards the end of the service I spent a week-end on the farm, and at night in my sleep I wakened Alice by trying to empty her breasts. This so alarmed the family that I was not allowed to return to my nursing job.

In the fall of 1886 the money that I had earned while teaching in St. Louis had dwindled to a few dollars. Nevertheless, I matriculated for the senior year, and would have entered college had I not received a message from Alice, who was teaching in Saginaw, Michigan. She wanted me to take a position made vacant by the sickness of one of their teachers. I would have to teach mathematics and German, and could live with her.

This was an alluring offer, and I accepted. The teaching was not difficult, and I found time to give massage to Dr. Freeman's patients. Dr. Freeman was the father of Alice Freeman Palmer, President of Wellesley College for many years.

The following spring, while still teaching, I learned that the position of demonstrator of anatomy in the University of Michigan Medical School was vacant. I applied, although I did not have my degree in medicine. Fortunately, my A.B. was accepted in lieu of the M.D. degree, and the position, carrying a salary of fifty dollars a month, was mine. This improvement in my financial condition, however, presented a problem of its own. How could I get enough knowledge of anatomy to fill the position? The only way out would be to go to Ann Arbor, and dissect all summer.

I spent every day from June till October in the dissecting room, rising at three in the morning, preparing breakfast for myself and E. C. Williams, one of my old literary as well as medical classmates, and dissecting from four till noon. The afternoon was devoted to study, and I retired soon after dinner.

There were six of us who dissected all summer. I shared my cadaver with a tall, pale, city-bred fellow who became easily tired and took frequent rests. Physical endurance has always been easy for me, and I could sit for hours, almost immovable, picking out bits of fat and separating the tissues, one from another. As my interest increased, my cheeks became redder until they vied with the color of my hair. I think it was this contrast between us that made my companions conjure up a theory that I was sapping the vitality of my side partner, and they took turns in making such remarks as these:

"Dodge, she's sapping your strength. You're compelled to rest more and more. Cut out the couch."

"You're getting weaker and weaker. Every day I see you frailing."

"Look, Dodge, she never gets tired and she never rests. She grows stronger all the time."

My medical degree, hard as I had worked for it and as much as I valued it, brought me no sense of competency. Responsibility for the life of a patient frightened me. I was different from my classmates who were eager to begin practice. When I insisted that I would like to work in a hospital for a time, they laughed at me and said, "I can't afford it."

Internships and residencies were in their incipiency and not popular with the student body. Tortured by a medical-practice inferiority complex, I applied to the Woman's Hospital in Detroit for a residency, and the Board of Trustees, appreciating my strenuous services during the summer as medical-student nurse, appointed me for the coming year.

Since I had to begin my residency one month before graduation, it was necessary to take special, private examinations in all senior subjects, but this gave me no concern, for Dr. Vaughn, in line with his customary treatment of women students, gave me credit without any examination beyond a few teasing remarks.

On the way to the anatomy examination I met a group of senior girls who began quizzing me. "Can you name the foramina in the petrous portion of the temporal bone?"

"In a final, such questions are foolish and unfair," I retorted. At this, they glibly rolled off the answer to it, and to two other equally finical questions.

To my amazement the anatomy teacher asked only those three

questions, and to his amusement I poured forth the answers with breathless fluency lest in another minute I should have forgotten them.

Listening to courses the required second time, attending operations that were performed in the surgical clinic without antiseptic precautions, and at the same time demonstrating anatomy to earn a living kept me busy; and it seemed a short time before they pronounced us ready to graduate.

Just before the graduation date, I was approached to contribute toward the purchase of a black silk dress for a woman student who had worked her way through school.

"Yes, yes," I quickly handed out my assessment, "and is every girl who has put herself through college going to receive a silk dress? You know I am a worthy candidate."

"You're different," came the reply, which compensated for having to make with my own hands, a graduating dress out of one of my old ones.

Perhaps I was different. On the farm I had learned how to meet realities without suffering either mentally or physically. My initiative had never been blunted. I had freedom to succeed—freedom to fail. Life on the farm produces a kind of toughness.

PRACTICE MAKES PERFECT

WHEN PEOPLE ask me why I consider training quite as important as theory, I tell this story.

Dr. John Dill Robinson, the Chicago Commissioner of Health who took smoking out of the city's streetcars and elevated trains, organized some short lecture courses in nursing shortly after the influenza epidemic of 1918.

Mature and intelligent women were admitted to these lectures and after three months of concentrated daily instruction were placed with physicians for a little practical application of what they had learned. One of these women, while assisting a physician with a wound dressing, saw the sterile dressing fall to the floor. She started to pick it up, then hesitated, a puzzled frown on her face.

Suddenly her expression cleared. Pointing to the fallen dressing she said "You pick it up, Doctor," adding knowingly, "you're more sterile than I am!"

9

FOUR YEARS WITH OBSTETRICS, INSANITY, AND SURGERY

WHEN I BEGAN service in the Woman's Hospital, Detroit, my predecessor had left four post partum patients, one delivered two days previously, and the other three patients, several weeks before. All had fever and were being given hot vaginal douches three times a day. The day I arrived, the patient most recently delivered had a chill and became acutely ill. The first two cases I delivered had chills and fever on the third and fourth days.

I had been on duty two weeks before it dawned on me that every patient in the hospital had childbed fever! I had to face the grim fact—an epidemic of puerperal fever!

Forty years before, in 1843, Dr. Oliver Wendell Holmes had pointed out that the cause of childbed fever was contagion. In 1847, Semmelweis, in Vienna, attributed the disease to the introduction of decomposing animal matter into the vagina, insisting that if the obstetrician or midwife would wash the hands in chlorine water before delivering the woman, epidemics could be prevented. His hidebound medical colleagues treated his revolutionary research with such distrust and such contumely that, disheartened, he became demented and died without receiving the recognition due him as the savior of mothers.

In the seventies, Lister brought forth and applied the germ theory to everyday problems, and Semmelweis was resurrected while his associates slept on in the cemetery of obstructionists. In the brief period of twenty years following Lister's research, students were taught that the physician and nurses were responsible for fever after delivery.

Accepting the disgrace, I called upon the shades of my Dutch ancestors to direct me until all was "clean as blood of babes." I aired, scrubbed, boiled and soaked in bichloride of mercury solution, the sheets, mattresses, beds, walls, floors, and the patients' and doctors' gowns. I did this not once—but day after day, for there were no rooms for segregating patients, and the nurse and I cared for both fresh deliveries and old infected ones.

It was a strenuous, not to say exhausting fight. I was so wearied as well as worried, that I feared that I might, like Semmelweis, become demented. During those weeks, as soon as I fell asleep, I would see at the foot of my bed four tall coffins standing on end. On each coffin plate was the name of the patient, and below it the significant information, "Doctored by Bertha Van Hoosen." This dream was so real and impeaching that it would invariably awaken me, and slipping out of bed, I would revisit the ward to reassure myself that the patients were not in coffins standing on end, and that I was not behind bars.

No patient died, and after the first month none developed fever. I have never regretted that harrowing experience, for I learned what could be done to prevent infection, even under the most discouraging circumstances.

With one exception I had been able to conduct all of the deliveries without calling upon the visiting staff. My last case, however, proved to be a Jonah. She was a mentally-deficient girl, Cyclopean, with double thumbs on each hand, and six toes on each foot. I had not anticipated trouble with her delivery, but the girl lived up to her anomalous physical structure by furnishing the most pathological delivery in the history of the hospital.

The huge creature was like a patient animal in her reaction to pain, but after many hours the labor showed no progress. The baby's head rested high above the pelvis, and only a small portion of it was wedged into the inlet as the result of the driving force of the pains. The foetal heart was good and the mother easily controlled, but I began to worry about the advisability of calling for assistance.

Once before I had been obliged to call one of the attending obstetricians to deliver a patient who had a small tumor obstructing the birth canal. Dr. Flinterman answered the call, and after making an examination, asked me to apply forceps.

At that time I had hesitated, for my knowledge of forceps had been obtained entirely from books.

"All right, watch me." With enviable skill and celerity he applied the tong-like instruments, and then, to my astonishment, instead of delivering the baby he slipped the forceps off and said, "Now you apply them."

I had succeeded fairly well, but as I turned for his approval, he again removed the instruments with, "You will feel more at home; try again."

I wonder how many lives that wonderful lesson by a truly great master has saved in the past half century.

Yes, I must call again for assistance. But just when? If too early, I ran the chance of being ridiculed and mortified by facetious remarks about over-solicitous women physicians. Too late, and I become responsible for a death, perhaps two deaths.

Preferring to suffer ridicule rather than the torments of a guilty conscience, I called Dr. Longyear. He was a handsome gentleman, very courteous and kind, but he made me feel inferior because I was a woman—an irremediable condition.

With mannerly condescension he asked me to apply the instruments, at the same time making the comforting remark that the patient had certainly had a fair chance to show what she could do for herself. The application of the forceps was more difficult than in the case where I had called Dr. Flinterman—dear, rough and ready Dr. Flinterman, how grateful I was to him!—but all went well, and I applied the forceps successfully. The situation took on a more hopeful aspect, and grasping firmly the handles of the forceps, I made gentle traction. Again and again I made traction.

When I realized that my efforts were availing nothing, my spirits began to droop, but I was determined to bring that baby. Failure after failure to dislodge the head urged me to redouble my exertion. My strength was slowly waning. My hands were visibly trembling. My legs were shaking. (Thank God for petticoats!) I could no longer hang on to the forceps. Like a knocked-out pugilist, I was down.

Dr. Longyear scrutinized me with sympathetic superiority and remarked, "I guess it needs a little masculine muscle."

I agreed faintly as he handled the forceps gracefully and expertly, and made gentle traction, which was repeated and repeated, each time with more and more force. He was covered with perspiration and his hands, too, were shaking. Finally, glancing at me, he gasped, "Well, well, we will have to have more help. Send for Dr. Carsten."

Dr. Carsten came, but he only duplicated our efforts.

In an atmosphere of desperate gloom Dr. Longyear asked me to put my arms under those of the patient, and pull at the same time that both he and Dr. Carsten, uniting their strength, pulled on the forceps. He was determined to deliver the baby! Unsuccessful and discouraged, the two doctors sat down, steaming from their great exertion.

The only course left was to dismember the baby, and deliver it piecemeal. How distasteful this mutilating operation, performed on an ordinary bed, in the patient's room and with a minimum of untrained assistants, must have been to Dr. Carsten, the most skillful woman's surgeon in Detroit! Even so, he did not waver, and soon I saw a slender stream of brains exuding from the vagina. Then came lungs and intestines, next arms, and finally the dismembered body. For days the mother hovered between life and death, and weeks were consumed in the repair of the injured tissues and recovery from shock.

At this time the Woman's Hospital received only delinquent girls, but none of them was of the prostitute type, and most of them came from "good families". Some entered the institution early in pregnancy, while others were residents for only a short time before delivery. It was the rule, however, that no girl could be discharged until a satisfactory home had been found for the baby.

I was shocked when I first learned that the babies of all these unmarried mothers were adopted. On the farm it had distressed me when the new-born calves were separated from their mothers. Sleep was impossible when, all through the night, I heard the cows lowing for their babies. The horses and sheep were my balm in Gilead, for they were never separated from their young that nursed and frolicked all day long.

To calm my emotions, the matron and the chairman of the adoption committee assured me that when the girls kept their babies they usually found it so difficult to support them that eventually the babies were deserted or became victims of malnutrition. They were positive that the suffering of separation was only deferred.

Young and untutored in sociology, I tried to accept their system as best for all concerned, but every time I witnessed the modus operandi of an adoption, my doubts doubled.

My memory retains all the grim details of these baby-finding incidents. One sunny afternoon the sound of horses' hoofs and the roll of wheels was heard on the little-used approach to the hospital. Every girl heard the meaningful sound and made an excuse to get near a window or secret peephole. When the elegant carriage, with driver and footman and drawn by matched horses stopped, a lady of the gay nineties with bobbing bustle and waving plumes stepped out. The nursery matron circled importantly around the nursery, admonishing the mothers to dress their babies in their "prettiest" and then go to the wash room and wait for her. The lady was conducted to the nursery and invited, like a dinner guest, to "help yourself." She flitted and fluttered from one crib to another, unable to make a decision. She called upon the matron for assistance, but got none. Should it be the little girl with yellow curls or the boy with snapping black eyes? Just then a little fellow stretched out his arms to the childless woman. He was chosen. The lady was conducted back to the visitors' room, and the matron released the breathless girls huddled in the lavatory. "Well, Mary," she called, "you are a lucky girl. Your baby will have one of the finest homes in the country. Hurry, now, and dress him." She handed Mary a bag containing baby clothes so dainty and expensive that the girl was afraid to touch them. Slowly and tenderly, Mary slipped the tiny garments on her infant. Smoothing his blonde hair for a moment, she looked down to admire him cradled in her arms. Then the child slipped from her blurred vision. The matron caught the baby as its fainting mother fell to the floor.

I worked over Mary for an hour. She slowly regained consciousness and realization that now she was free to go back into the world, alone.

Some of these girls were emotionally more unstable than others. One, a Canadian, entered the hospital when she was near the end of her pregnancy. She had been starving herself for months, and a few days after her delivery she became insane. This form of insanity that attacks women after their delivery is known as puerperal and often lasts for several months. In the case of this patient the cause was, without doubt, her exhausted physical condition. Although not especially difficult to manage she had decided infanticidal and suicidal tendencies, and had to be watched constantly.

I was with her so much that I felt acquainted, through listening to her ravings, with the undertaker, a married man, father of her baby. I could almost hear the words of her stern English father as he denounced any unmarried girl who became a mother. I actually shed tears for his timid, self-effacing wife who dared not help her daughter in the time of her great need. Sometimes in her delirium she would spend the entire night with her ranting father and sobbing mother. Towards morning her father would seem to have crushed her, and muttering, "I'll have to do it," she would fall asleep with a piece of torn sheet wound many times around her neck.

At other times her frenzied conversation was with her lover.

She would plead piteously with him to do something for her, to take her life or to give her poison so that she might die.

To me the most distressing hours were when she would attempt to kill the baby. She would seize a pillow, rock it in her arms, kissing and caressing it. Then with staring eyes and clenched teeth she would squeeze and squeeze the soft resisting sack until her hands fell limp and her breath was spent.

It was six weeks after the baby had been born before she regained her mental health, and I was surprised that her mania did not deprive her of her courage and good sense. She returned to her native town, able to meet the world and start a new life, for her insane experiences had left no record in her brain.

I needed and enjoyed every minute of my obstetrical residency, but when I was urgently invited to return to Ann Arbor to demonstrate anatomy during the winter months, I left the Woman's Hospital, with its perplexing problems of delinquent girls and their beautiful, bastard babies, without a regret.

I was glad to return to the dissecting room. It was never a gruesome place to me. While sitting in silent communion with my cadaver, I felt the presence of the Divine Architect of man more keenly than when I entered a church.

In the spring, as the anatomy course was nearing an end, Dr. Mary Black Palmer who had been assistant physician at the Kalamazoo State Hospital before she married its superintendent, urged me to fill the vacancy which she had recently made.

I had always had an unreasoning fear of insane people. Once, during my college days, everyone rushed to the window to see an insane man who had taken off all his clothes, painted his body with indigo and climbed into a leafless tree. I did not join the curious crowd. The lunatic terrified me so that I fled through the back door, climbed a wire fence, stayed away from dinner, and worried a great deal lest I might catch sight of such a wild, strange creature.

Dr. Black Palmer was unable to persuade me to take the position. She talked a long time and finally proposed that if I would come and stay a month, I would not need to do any work, and I would be paid twenty-five dollars. This was such an absurd offer, and so unusual after I had been counting dollars and cents for five years, that I at last accepted, feeling much like a joker in a pack.

I occupied a beautiful suite of rooms with bath, and ate with Dr. Black Palmer and her husband. Every day I had fresh flowers from the conservatory, rode with the doctors in a comfortable carriage behind a spanking team, played tennis in the afternoon and whist in the evening. At the end of the month I was five pounds heavier and twenty-five dollars richer.

This life was nearer to that of royalty and the millionaire class than anything I have experienced since. Nevertheless, I began to want a hospital position with a regular salary. After a talk with Dr. Palmer, the superintendent, this was arranged. I was to receive a salary of seventy-five dollars a month for special care of the insane women patients, and medical charge of some wards.

My first duty was to look after new patients, and record any marks or bruises found on the body. The first examination I made necessitated passing through a convalescent ward (that was easy), a mildly-disturbed ward (that was worse), and then into the violent ward, where the new patient was being bathed. Trembling and breathless with fear, I reached the patient, observed her, and then dreaded the trip back to the office. I would have gladly climbed out the window or escaped by the roof. Instead, I must retrace my steps through wards that were filled with the patients of whom I had such fear. When I was in the middle of the mildly-disturbed ward, I heard running feet behind me. My heart stood still—I tried to scream, but could not—I could not even move my head—it was like a nightmare. Nearer and nearer the running steps came; then a heavy slap on my back, a whisper in my ear, "Who are you?" Before I could see my assailant, she had fled out of sight, but she took with her all my fears. No insane patient has ever frightened me since.

Dr. Palmer, who was years in advance in the care of the insane and in institutional management, taught me many things outside of the field of medicine. He personally instructed me how to inspect wards, dining rooms, and bathrooms; he took forks and ran a fold of cloth between the tines; he lifted the drinking glasses to the light and squinted for lint; he traced a figure eight with his finger on the bottom of the dishpan, looking for grease. In the wards, standing on a chair, he passed his hand over the partitions between the windowpanes.

There were no restraints applied to patients, and no special nurses assigned to suicidal or homicidal cases. After the addition of a new building at the Pontiac State Hospital many of the patients from our overcrowded hospital in Kalamazoo were transferred. The young physician who came for them asked, "Which ones are suicidal, and need special nurses?"

Dr. Palmer explained, "None has a special nurse. All sleep in a ward, and are never alone. Given plenty of time, people will always put off doing things, even to committing suicide."

Instead of accepting this hypothesis, the young man, as soon as he had returned with his charges, placed two special nurses on one of the worst cases. A week later the patient committed suicide, although she had made no such attempt in many years in Kalamazoo. Her suicide was accomplished by jumping upon a chair and falling backward, breaking her neck. She did this in the few minutes while the nurses chatted during the interchange of duty.

While in the Kalamazoo State Hospital, I was the only woman on the staff with seven men, and so became the natural butt of a practical joke. I was informed that every Friday it was my duty to go to the dispensary and extract the teeth of any patients who had been sent there.

I had never pulled a tooth in my life and never expected to, but though scared to death, I determined not to give up unless I failed. My first patient had pyorrhoea, and wanted me to pull all of her teeth. They almost fell out, and my confidence was so restored that I was soon enjoying the job.

I had extracted about a thousand teeth before the superintendent discovered what was going on. It seemed it was the druggist's duty to do this work, but I baffled the conspirators and voluntarily continued to pull teeth as long as I remained there.

Not a year has passed since that time, more than fifty years ago, when I have not mulled over the case of Mary Jane. She was under the special care of one of the attending doctors who force-fed her five times a day. Occasionally, when he was away, I pushed the long stomach tube down the gullet of the unresisting Mary Jane, and the nurse poured into the connecting funnel a pint of rich, liquid nourishment.

Here is a layman's abstracted history of the case: Before Mary Jane became a patient in an insane hospital, she had had a delightful courtship, a short engagement and, deliriously happy, was dressed in bridal finery for her wedding. The guests had assembled, and everything was in readiness except one very essential thing—the bridegroom.

As she sat on her bed waiting for the arrival of her belated fiance, a letter was handed to her. She opened it, read the enclosed note, but made no sign to move. One of her bridesmaids, fretting at the delay, glanced over her shoulder and saw these lines, "I love you too much to go on with this. I am already married."

From that moment until I saw her six months after her entrance into the asylum, Mary Jane had never voluntarily moved, never lifted her head or swallowed, even her saliva that drizzled down over her chin. She could be moved by being pushed about like a dummy, and dressed as a child dresses a doll.

One day, while substituting for the regular physician, I found the attendants greatly excited over Mary Jane who, upon hearing someone say, "The boy stood on the burning deck," snapped back, "Whence all but him had fled."

They repeated the first line of every jingle and ditty they could recall and Mary Jane responded by reciting the second line.

A little later Mary Jane began to walk, but no one could inveigle her into stepping on the red stripe in the long hall runner. When she came to the red, it seemed to be a danger signal, and with both feet she jumped over it.

Three times a day Mary Jane had been taken to the dining

room, although she never even looked at the table or moved her hands. But, after she began to talk and walk, she added to these accomplishments that of eating her dinner at the table with the other patients.

Then came the big surprise for us. Mary Jane had become quite normal in every way. She knew the content of the fateful letter and was grateful to have been spared a bigamous marriage, but remembered nothing that had happened from the day she read it until after she had been in the asylum the best part of a year. However, she did remember and rehearsed in lip-smacking detail everything that her physician had said to the head nurse during the frequent, daily feeding periods. The doctor was in love with the nurse, and their pretty talk must have had a lovely response when fresh, but when recited in a flat voice by Mary Jane, it afforded better amusement than any other offering in Kalamazoo.

Mary Jane never tired of broadcasting "The Private Affairs of the Doctor and the Head Nurse," and I have always believed that it was the daily reiteration of endearing love, more than the forced feeding that wakened the shocked and dormant centers in Mary Jane's brain and brought her back to life. She made a complete recovery and was discharged a well and surprisingly happy woman.

After a three-months' study of patients I was convinced that many were not insane at all, but before my service was over, I had many demonstrations of my faulty diagnosis.

My first awakening was when the lovely old gentleman who worked in the library and regularly took the horse and buggy to get the mail for the institution, did not appear. He had started for the post office, but when hours passed and he did not return, scouts were sent out. He was discovered, sitting by the roadside, pounding his very valuable watch, an heirloom, to bits, while the horse patiently cropped the roadside grass. After some weeks of violence he again appeared the same courteous, reliable, delightful person that I had thought to be perfectly well.

Another was a fine, young college-educated man whom I had

known at Ann Arbor. I could see nothing wrong with his mental health. Nevertheless, one morning he went to the carpenter shop where he was working and, before anyone was aware of what he was doing, he had chopped off his penis with a sharp hatchet—his solution to annoying sex problems.

While in the Woman's Hospital in Detroit, I had been an eye witness to what, at the time, I thought to be the worst of physical and mental pain, but after a few months at the Kalamazoo Insane Hospital I regarded the suffering of those unmarried mothers as ephemeral and perhaps chastening.

I came to look upon insanity as a living death more than a disease—a living death like that suffered by those damned souls in the concentric circles of the inferno.

With such a feeling I often visited a sweet, delicate little lady whose delusion was that she was dead. She thought that anything which would kill another person could not harm her because she was already dead. She was so obsessed with this idea that very rarely would she stop talking about being dead long enough for me to introduce a more pleasant subject.

If I wore a hat, she would beg me to take my hat pin and thrust it deeply into her heart. "That would kill anybody, wouldn't it? Try it on me; run it into my heart. It will not kill me." At other times she begged me to choke her for fifteen minutes. "That would kill anybody except me. I am already dead; it will not kill me." She was constantly conjuring up some new and fantastic method for producing death and urging everyone she met to try it on her.

She occupied a pleasant room on the convalescent floor, but her companions, though insane themselves, regarded her as a "boresome nut." Her husband came frequently to take her for a drive. On one of these occasions she seemed so like her normal self that instead of hitching the horse and accompanying her back to her room, he allowed her, at her earnest request, to return alone. It was not long before the nurses missed her. Search was instituted and her decapitated body was found, lying on the railroad track that ran back of the asylum.

In medical school I received no instruction in psychiatry, and during my assistantship in the Kalamazoo Insane Hospital I did not acquire even a vocabulary in that subject. Whenever female patients were admitted to the institution, I examined them for evidence of any physical injury such as cuts, scars, burns or bruises, but made no other examinations.

During my eighteen months' service I never made a note on the mental or physical condition of any patient, except in an occasional letter to their relatives. These letters were subjected to the approval of the superintendent, who had instructed me in the use of phrases that could not be used in court against the institution or the staff. I became expert in expressing myself in such terms as: "If your sister continues in her present condition, I see no reason why your anxiety concerning her should be more than what you naturally feel."

In the nineteenth century, treatment for the insane was little more than confinement (occasionally with restraints), a regular routine of living, employment, amusement, occasional doses of castor oil and an iron tonic. Brain surgery, physiotherapy, shock treatment, psychoanalysis as well as vitamin and endocrine medication were later developments.

The training of nurse attendants was exceptionally fine and was largely responsible for the improvement and recovery of many cases. On every occasion they were found to be unflinching soldiers with but one thought—the discharge of duty.

As a conspicuous example of their courage, one day one of our best trained nurse attendants, while making rounds, stooped to button the collar of a very untidy patient. Just as she finished, the patient lowered her head, caught the last joint of the nurse's index finger between her teeth, and with a single clamp of the jaw bit the end off.

Without a word, the nurse picked up the amputated part of the finger as it rolled upon the floor, took it to the office and asked the doctor if he could restore it. Unfortunately, it was impossible to do so, but on the following day all of the patient's front teeth were extracted.

The sacrifices made and the dangers daily encountered by these nurse attendants in caring for the insane should receive not only recognition, but the deepest gratitude from the public.

The fearlessness and self-control of these young women stimulated me to do many things that before entering into the service of the insane I would have thought impossible. As the only woman on the staff, I was frequently asked to try my hand at coaxing from her lair a wild patient who periodically barricaded the door of her room with her bed, bureau and other furniture. No one could enter, nor would she come out.

When I was asked to try my hand at breaking into her stockade, I was given carte blanche to use any method that might assist me in bringing forth the self-imprisoned lady.

Perfectly aware that it would require time and no end of patience, I armed myself with the key to the door of the general storehouse and a low chair. Seating myself so that my mouth came on a level with the keyhole, I released a program of masterful seduction. I opened with pleasantries about her health and the weather. She replied in the language of a drunken pirate. I invited her to take a walk. I handed out interesting bits of ward gossip, and at the end of an hour I succeeded in persuading her to remove the blockade sufficiently for me to enter the room. Even so, the moment I was inside, as per agreement, the furniture was replaced against the door.

As I looked around the room, I found that she had smeared the walls, as high as her long, skinny arms could reach, with her bowel excreta, and that the atmosphere was nauseating with the abhorrent odor.

Now that I was her prisoner, I bent all my energies to interest her in the things that we might discover if we made a visit to the general storehouse. In many tempting ways I displayed the key that was in my possession. At last she listened. Like a genuine burglar pal I whispered my plan: we would slip out of the room and secretly visit the storehouse. Once there, we would possess ourselves of everything we fancied. Although she was interested, another hour passed before she seriously considered leaving her room. Then, on tiptoe, we warily crept through the door into the long hall and down the back stairs where patients were never allowed. Crouching against the building, we moved cautiously until we reached our goal—the storehouse with its wealth of merchandise of every description.

After entering, I locked the door behind us and left my patient to her own devices. She was soon lost in the delights of looting. Over her tangled and graying hair, she tried on hat after hat. She forced her bare feet into all sizes and kinds of shoes. She held up one dress and then another against her corsetless gangling frame. Fingering through piles of towels, sheets, curtains and men's clothing, she seemed unable to decide on anything that she would like to possess. Her freedom to act and the riches before her satiated all her cravings. When at last she settled upon one bright-colored handkerchief, her next desire was to return to the ward and display it before the other patients.

With no arguments on my part or resistance on hers, we hurried back and found that the nurses had cleaned and restored her chamber to the faultlessly appointed order of all asylum rooms.

I had spent three hours with this mad woman, but I had the satisfaction of having saved a posse of men from the dangers of physical injury from broken glass and flying furniture. A wild fight in all probability would have been the result if they had entered her room through the transom and taken her by force.

I had been in Kalamazoo more than a year when I had typhoid fever, with two relapses, carrying a very high temperature for nine weeks, and in coma the last. Just before the attack, while eating a hearty dinner with my colleagues in the asylum dining room, I made the remark, "People should not fear death. I myself have absolutely no fear of death."

At that one of the assisting physicians, Dr. Tullidge, whose father was a Presbyterian minister, said, "Don't ever make such a remark as that again. You don't know what you are talking about, sitting there the picture of health. It sounds absurd."

"Well, I cannot prove it today, but I may some day."

After leaving the table, I felt chilly and could not get warm though I stood in front of a hot radiator until the keys in my hand almost burned me. Finally, I went to bed, and was lying smothered under seven blankets, when Dr. Black Palmer found me and took my temperature. It was one hundred and seven. I was delirious.

When the doctor who had been appointed to take charge of my case, visited me, I would plead day after day, "Tell Dr. Tullidge that I am not afraid to die." Or, "Why didn't you let me die yesterday? I am not afraid." I proved my point, though I nearly lost my life as well as all of my hair doing it.

Shortly after my phenomenal recovery from typhoid, I learned that the New England Hospital for Women and Children was looking for a resident. The application had to be made in person. Life in the well-managed insane institution was so easy and luxurious that I worried about its ultimate effect on me. So I turned my back on its allurements and set out for Boston, stopping at Montclair, New Jersey, to visit Alice, who had just returned from her honeymoon in England.

I had made all of my own dresses, and was concerned only about my professional ability. Alice said at once, "You will never get the place unless you buy yourself some new clothes."

She took me to McAlpin's in New York, where I was fitted out with a diagonal-striped wool dress with a basque of the same material, and leg-of-mutton sleeves of plain brown silk. The skirt was very long, sweeping the ground, with a silk ruffle a foot wide. Then I bought an astrachan pelerine, and a hat covered with wings, suggesting a flight of birds—a remarkable fashion but no stranger than some of our "Candy-kid" creations. My hair, that had not grown long since my typhoid, was a mass of short red curls.

As a Western woman with limited clinical experience, I had little hope of being the successful candidate. There was only one other applicant, and she was well fitted for the position, but the board of medical women who made the selection liked my personal appearance. Confidentially, I had feared my fine feathers would militate against me, for the Boston medical women were dressed in clothes that were at least four years out of date.

Later, I learned that the choice narrowed down to two points: hair and training. My hair was short from force of circumstances and my opponent's, from choice. In addition, I had a wider training in obstetrics, a necessary qualification for the position.

When I began my service, I had no idea of what would be expected of me, but I soon found out. My duties consisted of seeing every patient in the hospital at least once a day; doing one-third of the surgical operations and assisting in the others; conducting all abnormal deliveries; keeping a daybook; attending the private clinic twice a week; and last but not least, being responsible for the teaching and deportment of six interns—a big program under the best of circumstances, but more difficult because I was suffering from an inferiority complex that was not without foundation.

Soon after my arrival, one of the attending staff on the medical service advised, "Now Dr. Van Hoosen, I want to give you some hints. Our surgeons will cheat you out of doing any surgery if you don't mind your p's and q's. Insist on your rights! There's a ruling that the resident shall do one-third of the operations, but when I was resident, I never got any to do. Now, you see to it that you don't get cheated."

I was too overpowered with my responsibilities to let this make any impression upon me, and I notified Dr. Mary Smith, who was nearing the end of a three-month surgical service, "I wish to act as an assistant for at least a month, or until I have learned the hospital routine."

The month passed quickly, when another physician, Dr. Keller, came on surgical service. I assisted her with two very simple operations, but the third was on a woman with lacerations suffered twenty years previously in childbirth. This patient had no control of the bowels, and her operation, if successful, must result in normal bowel action.

When Dr. Keller asked in the most casual manner, "Would you like to do the operation?" I thought how absurd it was to think that these women surgeons would cheat me out of my rightful opportunity. On the contrary, they were showing perfect fairness.

Determined to make myself worthy of their confidence, I assured Dr. Keller, "I will be very glad, with your help, to do the operation."

That night I studied till long after midnight on the anatomy and surgery of the perineum. With a fresh, vivid picture of the intricately woven muscles and fascia that make up that small structure, I mentally repaired, not once, but many times, those lacerations that had undergone scar retraction and muscle atrophy.

In the morning I rose early, trying not to be nervous and excited. At seven-thirty (the operation was scheduled sharply at eight) Dr. Keller telephoned me, "I will not be able to come to the hospital this morning; but you go right ahead with the operation."

I was stunned by her faith in my ability, and vowed that it would never be let down, that I would show myself worthy. If it had been a less formidable operation, it would not have been such a demonstration of her confidence in me! I must make good!

As luck—yes, luck—would have it, the operation proved a success, but the success of the surgery did not impress me so much as the fact that I had not failed the trust placed in me.

The fourth and fifth were very minor operations, but the sixth was a cancer of the right breast. Dr. Keller, in exactly the same casual tone, asked, "Would you like to do the operation?"

With the deepest gratitude and a fierce determination not to disappoint her, I again accepted the opportunity offered and dug into the anatomy and surgery of the breast until the small hours of the morning.

This time Dr. Keller was there to assist. I took off the breast, and started to remove the glands from under the arm when Dr. Keller suggested leaving them.

I handed the knife over to her, admitting, "I will probably

not do it so rapidly or so well as you, but," with sharp emphasis, "the glands must be removed."

She did not accept the knife, but directed, "Proceed!"

During my service at the Woman's Hospital in Detroit, I had become so interested in the problems of illegitimate offspring that when I took over the residency at the New England Hospital the first question I asked was, "Where are the unmarried mothers and their babies?"

Miss Clark, one of the James Freeman Clark family and chairman of the Committee for Delinquent Girls, responded cheerfully, "Oh, we always find places for them to work in the country where they can take their babies, and they usually marry sons of the neighboring farmers, often the sons of the family for whom they are working."

"But," I remonstrated, "what about the girl's reputation and the stigma attached to the child?"

Miss Clark smiled. "Reputation is not of enough value to sacrifice character for it."

I became a vocal convert.

10

A HOME DELIVERY

NEARLY FOUR YEARS of hospital training had a marked effect upon my medical ego. I found on completing my service at the New England Hospital for Women and Children that I had become hypercritical of the work of staff physicians, and was becoming self-confident to an alarming degree.

At long last I was in heat for private practice, and would have begun at once had not Alice entrusted to me a precious secret, "I'm going to have a baby."

To my query, "When?" she responded, "In June, I think."

June....

We realized our lives had suddenly undergone a tremendous transformation. Things would never again be the same.... Fear, hope, joy—a tumult of emotions almost choked me.

Up to her thirtieth year Alice had devoted her time to study and teaching, but the year after I graduated from medicine, she had changed her vocation and entered the medical department of the University of Michigan, where she had taken her A.B. degree seven years before.

During her years of teaching she had saved money in anticipation of a trip to Europe. The opportunity came during the summer of her junior year in medicine, and it was her maiden voyage in more senses than one, for she returned a bride.

Joseph Comstock Jones, at the time he married Alice, was head of the Educational Department of Harper & Brothers Publishers, which was the height of his ambition. When Harper & Brothers discontinued publishing school books two years later it was a staggering blow, for it meant that he must look for another position.

So it came to pass that Alice and Joe had planned to go to the farm in Stony Creek, Michigan, where Father and Mother were, and remain till Joe could find a job suited to his qualifications. I readjusted my plans that I might be with Alice at this crucial time, and take a much-needed rest before choosing a location for beginning private practice.

That Alice, Joe, and I should be going to the farm for an indefinite stay with Father and Mother seemed, with the prospect of the coming baby, to be nothing less than predestined fortune. That circumstances should enable the new baby to share the ancestral home, the birthplace of my mother, my sister, and me, was as much a miracle as birth itself.

Stony Creek seemed an ideal spot in which to begin life, especially embryonic life. Here a microscopic human egg, lying on its vascular bed, ought to be able, without interference, to divide and subdivide, to roll itself into layer upon layer, to bend and turn, to take on function and to become a being like those from whom it filched its chromosomes. I hoped that in this quiet hamlet Alice could have the assistance and brooding care of nature to bring to perfection an heir to the Stony Creek modest homestead.

That I should deliver her baby was a presupposed fact. Had I not been studying for the past twelve years to fit myself to take this precious responsibility? If I never did anything more, all the years spent in preparation were well employed in the light of what I might be able to do for Alice.

By spending four years getting my A.B. degree, four years in medical study, and finally, four years in hospital service, I had trebled the requirements made at that time by the medical school from which I had my degree.

The good doctors under whom I had interned in Detroit would be glad to help me if needed. That Alice might go to a hospital never occurred to us. In 1892 the Woman's Hospital in Detroit received only delinquent girls as patients, and home deliveries were the vogue. There was a marked difference between the obstetric attitude in the nineteenth century, when all deliveries were adjudged normal, and in this twentieth century, when any delivery may suddenly be considered abnormal.

The present popular prenatal care was in embryonic state in 1892, but its principles were recognized and taught in medical schools: fresh air, especially country air, fresh foods—comprising milk, eggs, fruit and vegetables—housework, furnishing exercise of great variety, and frequent opportunities to rest—in fact all of the conditions promoting the normal functions of the body. The necessity for the examination of the urine was well understood in those days.

Alice was in excellent general health, with none of the morbid symptoms that so many women experience. She had had no vomiting, not even nausea, no annoyance or fright from movements of the child and no signs of dropsical swelling, hemorrhoids, or urinary disturbances—none of a host of woes that befall many expectant mothers.

She did a great deal of housework, almost too much, a girlhood habit, and found it irksome to sit and sew. When she relegated the making of the layette to me, I was as happy as a little girl with a new doll.

I was determined to make the clothes modern, hygienic, comfortable, sensible, scientific, but above all, attractive, and turned to good account my latent maternal instincts, my recently-acquired medical knowledge, and my aptitude for the manual arts.

The long, voluminous baby robe was beginning to be outmoded, and I went to the other extreme, making the dresses just to the legs, covering only the body. The baby's clothing consisted of a little shirt, a diaper, and this abbreviated dress.

A most important article was the papoose pillow whereby the baby could be tucked safely into a portable feather bed. The pillow was narrow, but long enough to fold back, leaving only the baby's arms and head exposed. The folded end was held securely by strings tied over it, and the pillow slips as well as strings were trimmed with ruffles.

I took pride in having everything handmade: diapers, embroidered blankets, bibs, and even a tiny bonnet. The pillow and the ballet baby dresses were the wonder and admiration of the village, and now, after fifty years, I still believe this outfit ideal for the newborn.

Even though Joe and I were jobless, the atmosphere of the home was happy. Many times I had heard Father say when some delinquent boy or girl had been turned from home, "My girls can do nothing so vile that the doors of my house would be closed to them. Just as long as I have a home, it is their home." If Alice or I had had a deed to the farm, and Father and Mother had been living with us, we could not have felt any more at home.

So the waiting days grew into weeks, the anxious weeks passed into months, until, at long last, on a rare June morning, Alice said, "I have a pain, not severe. It soon goes, but soon returns."

Then the birth watch began.

Joe was much older than Alice—a man fifty years of age, tall and straight as an Indian, with a walk that few men could imitate. His hair was white and served as a setting for his large, brown, tender eyes. A small goatee concealed a deep dimple in his chin, and gave a touch that harmonized with his incomparable and agile, shapely legs.

Yet, that day he looked years older, for he was anticipating impending danger. Little wonder, for this was his fourth experience in having a baby. My sister was his second wife, and the first wife's first baby had been born dead. With the birth of his third baby, both wife and baby had succumbed.

Nevertheless, there was a smile on his face as he endeavored to make the time pass pleasantly by taking Alice to a seat on the porch and reading to her or talking over a book that he had read.

I realized too keenly that we might encounter storms, for this was a first baby, and Alice was thirty-five years of age. Therefore, I did not try to shorten this period of calm.

During my residency in the Woman's Hospital in Detroit and the New England Hospital for Women and Children in Boston, I had attended and delivered many women, and could visualize every page of travailology. I had been with laboring women from the first annoying discomfort to their final catastrophic release, so sudden that the long strain and tension gave way to chattering teeth and shaking limbs.

I had been a witness to their cheerful courage when the long-awaited signs appeared. I had admired their determination to be brave, and willingness to pay the price of motherhood though it might be great.

I had returned their smiles until pain took the speech from their mouths and brought profound silence. I had helped them when they sought relief by walking and clinging to furniture, until, losing control, they threw themselves upon the bed, burning tears streaming down their cheeks.

The intense suffering had shocked me when women in labor cast aside all conventionalities, and grasped anything or anyone, with the ferocity of birds of prey, crying out and begging piteously for help, "Give me something, anything! Give me poison! I cannot live! I cannot stand another pain! See how weak I am—I am dying—I am gone," over and over, repeating these appealing words until, exhausted, they lapsed into unconsciousness.

Their sleep brought comfort to me, but only for a few minutes, for the unbearable agony came surging back like a wave, leaping higher and higher until it broke into a foaming madness of despair.

I had stayed with them as hour after hour passed, and the pain did not lessen. Instead, each pain took on an increment in strength, each pain, an increment in length, until not only the patient was suffering and despairing but everyone within hearing suffered in sympathy with her.

When doubt and fear joined the watching, waiting group

that was asking, "Is everything all right? Can she stand the strain? How long must this keep up? Can't something be done to hasten the birth, or relieve the suffering?" I had come with reassurances and promises that it would not be long, maybe half an hour or maybe a little longer. I had seen the patient and her friends fix their attention on the clock as time passed.

When the patient, poor soul, as I had feared, had lost confidence in her doctor, in herself, in life, I girded myself not to yield to her pleas. "Doctor, it is already more than half an hour. Is it coming? Doctor, it's an hour! Isn't it coming soon? Doctor, it's three hours since you said it would come soon!"

Conscious of my professional duty, I wanted to allow the birth to take place normally. All entreaties must find me deaf and dumb.

Alice, having given up her medical study at the end of the junior year, could not share with me this lively picture of childbirth. She had had no practical obstetrical training, nor had she been interested in the sex life of the barnyard animals, having as a child been more with Mother, while I was always with Father.

Although she had no vivid conception of childbirth, she had, like my mother, an ability to meet emergencies, to endure pain and discomfort, and to pass through any and all vicissitudes with determination and resignation.

We had engaged a Woman's Hospital to make the ordeal more endurable, but my sense of responsibility was so overwhelming that I was immune to hunger, fatigue, or sleep—my whole being centered on Alice and her baby.

The labor began in the morning, continued all the afternoon, and though pains came regularly and forcefully, an examination indicated that this, the first stage of labor, was only initiated, and that it would be another twelve hours at least before birth could take place.

Alice was cheerful, uncomplaining, and I believed, hopeful. It was a great help to me that her confidence in my ability was complete. She seemed, in fact, to regard me as more than human.

There was so little that anyone could do at this stage that it seemed wise for everyone to lie down, and get as much rest as possible. I felt that I must see Alice every hour and listen to the baby's heart. With my ear on the abdomen I could hear the heart beats so strong and clear that the sound in itself was like a message from that inner world from whence the baby was to come, but where it lingered, loathe to leave.

As soon as I lay down, I fell asleep, but was glad to waken, for I had dreamed that I was at the Women's Hospital in Detroit, attending one of the delinquent girls in her first confinement. Every time I lapsed into sleep I dreamed of and lived over those harrowing deliveries of illegitimate children. Like a never-ending birth parade they passed through the hall of memory with a vividness of reality. The comforting thought came to me that abnormal deliveries were the exception, and that at times delivery did not occupy more than an hour or two. Since the beginning of Alice's labor I had rehearsed all of the deliveries I had ever seen or conducted and had increased my confidence.

It was still dark—just before the dawn. I closed my eyes, and particularized preparations for the delivery, which ought to take place sometime during the coming day. In the big dishpan I had ready: boiled forceps, a linen cord, a few needles and some silk sutures. I had chloroform and ergot, sterilized cotton and gauze, a bedpan, towels, a baby bathtub, and a solution of permanganate of potassium. This solution would be applied to my hands and arms until they were a dark mahogany color which was removed by scrubbing in a solution of oxalic acid. This procedure would take from fifteen to twenty minutes. I was confident I could conduct a delivery free from infection, for I had had a lesson in the hard school of experience.

The dawn seemed to be whipping everything into motion and life. Stepping to the long south porch, I saw on the horizon, in a crack between two buttock-rounded hills, a gleaming crescent tinted with crimson blood-like stain, rise and grow with momentary speed into a blushing head that led the way, till out of darkest night to Mother Earth was born a day. The birth was heralded by roosters crowing, cows mooing, barn doors swinging, and the appetizing smell of salt pork frying. It was the twenty-third of June! I thought at that time, and still think it was the most important June in my life. It was my niece's birthday.

Hoping that we might have that rare experience of a tedious labor suddenly becoming precipitous, everything was made ready for an emergency. Alice was looking tired. She had slept very little during the night, but at least she did not pass in review all of the abnormal cases in years of maternity service.

I listened more frequently to the baby's heart. It was good. The womb, however, had not opened enough to allow free passage for the baby. The labor had already consumed thirty hours, but it was still not possible to prognosticate the birth.

I was patient because I knew that in every birth the initial problem is to stretch a tiny hole scarcely large enough to admit a lead pencil until it will admit a baby's head. This stretching is accomplished by the intermittently contracting muscles of the womb pushing the baby's head against this little opening. In the course of an hour there may be fifteen to thirty contractions, and in thirty hours, at least five hundred. In this way the baby's head becomes molded from the shape of a ball to that of a sausage, and the tissues of the mother become soft and jelly-like. The hours crawled on until late afternoon.

The clock struck five as I listened to the baby's heart—what had happened? I listened again—there was no heart beat to be heard! "Quick, chloroform, drop by drop! Nurse!" Hastily, but with no difficulty the forceps were adjusted, and gentle traction made—how much I owed Dr. Flinterman! Through the narrow passage, with the aid of instruments, the baby moved, turned, and descended until the birth was checked only by the resistance of the skin at the outlet. The scissors quickly removed that barrier, and birth was allowed to take place, but it was a waxen baby that I saw. No piercing cry! Only a soggy, limp mass of non-palpitating protoplasm!

I held the baby by the feet, head downward. No sign of life!

Depressed spirits brought weariness, but not willingness to give up. Seated on the floor with my mouth pressed against the baby's, I sucked out the air, and then blew my own breath into those delicate lungs. For one-half hour this method of artificial respiration was continued without a sign of life in that pallid little form.

Joe came in and said, "The baby is dead. Anyone can see that. Please care for Alice. Don't let anything happen to her."

"Get out!" was my comforting response. Thirty-five minutes passed and nothing, not even a twitch of the tongue, gave evidence of life. Forty minutes—did I imagine it, or was there a slight fluttering over the heart?

I thought I felt a tremor in the tongue. Forty-five minutes—I was not deceived—a gasp—that was all I needed. Now I could work, unconscious of fatigue. Another gasp, one every minute, one every half-minute, oftener and oftener. A faint pink tint stole over the baby's body. The heart was visibly beating! The baby was breathing regularly! It was a girl—my little girl—for had I not breathed the breath of life into her when her own father said she was dead? And I—I wondered if God felt as I did when He created life!

Although the baby was breathing, she was cold in spite of the warm bath in which she was lying. Joe lighted the fire in the Franklin stove that had been set up in the adjoining sitting room.

"Get flannel clothes for us, Grandmother! Think of it—you are a grandmother!" I called to Mother.

With hot flannels, changed constantly, the little body gradually became warm. From seven in the evening until three the next morning I poured heat into her tiny body, as I had for one hour breathed air into her lungs. I wrapped her in her papoose pillow, and charted a new life.

A QUICK DIAGNOSIS

WHEN THE "snap diagnosis" spirit was in vogue, early in my practice, I was called to see a patient who had pain in her abdomen. I made a thorough and careful examination, but could not determine whether it was an attack of indigestion, an incipient appendicitis, or typhoid. I gave the patient a simple remedy that would not be contraindicated in any of the three possible diseases, and encouraged her with, "Don't be alarmed. You will be all right, and I will drop in tomorrow morning."

I reached for my hat, talking all the time so that the patient might not have an opportunity to ask me any questions—yet it was useless. She did not listen to my prattle, but fixing me with her eyes, demanded sharply, "What is the matter with me?"

If I told her I had the slightest suspicion of appendicitis, I knew she would send for another physician. If I said typhoid, and the next day she was well, she would think that I knew very little. And if I suggested it was nothing but indigestion, and it should prove to be appendicitis or typhoid, that would spell my doom. I resolved not to commit myself, so I replied cheerfully, "Why, you have rheumatism of the navel."

"Is that so?" She spoke very slowly and without smiling.

I lost no time in leaving. The patient was well the next day. No reference was made to the diagnosis.

11

SUBJECTS NOT TAUGHT IN MEDICAL SCHOOL

THE YEAR that my niece, Sarah, was born I selected a location and began the practice of medicine. This method of calendarizing happenings by "When Mabel had the mumps," or "Just after the twins were born," has a firm grip on me, though I have only the events in the life of this one niece for data from which to chart the polymorphic curve of my life.

In my career as in every one else's two questions were primary and essential—What? Where? The problem What? with all its uncertainties and ramifications was a thing of the past, and now I was face to face with Where?

My conception of a medical career at the age of eighteen had fructified. At long last I was a woman physician, hungry for professional contact with the world, but through my scientific knowledge, safe from its hazards.

The year on the farm, from the fall of 1891 to October, 1892, awaiting and attending Sarah's birth, served as a runway from which I could make a prudent take-off for my non-stop professional flight. Nonetheless, I spent many days, trying to make an unregrettable decision in solving the question Where?

Like all young people I was the possessor of countless theories, many of which, nipped by the frosts of experience, were doomed to inanition. My favorite hypothesis was, "Every hour brings light." This slogan was introduced to me in the senior year of my medical course when I sat at meals between two of my literary classmates, then studying for their Ph. D. degrees.

I remarked, one day, "I wish I could decide. . . ." whereupon Dr. Buckley spoke up, "Never waste time in decisions. Hough and I tried for a year not to make any decisions unless it was acutely necessary. Our slogan was, 'Every hour brings light.' During the year I made one decision and afterwards regretted it, but Hough never made one; when the decisive moment came, there was only one thing to do and he did it."

The whole United States might have had its arms outstretched to receive me, but my eyes were centered on four cities: St. Louis, Missouri, where Dr. Mary McLean had an affluent practice that she wished to share with me; Boston, Massachusetts, where I could have a position on the staff of the New England Hospital for Women and Children, and where I had already initiated a private practice through the privilege given the resident of a weekly pay clinic; Detroit, Michigan, where Father would pay my expenses until I was self-supporting, and where I had many acquaintances on the staff of the Woman's Hospital and in the city; and Milwaukee, Wisconsin, where my cousin, a surgeon, would refer to me all of his obstetric, pediatric, and medical cases.

Each one of these cities offered so many and such unusual advantages that, like the suitors before Portia's caskets, I hesitated lest I miss the prize.

Before casting the die, I thought it best to see Milwaukee. At this psychological moment Aunt Julia, the one who bribed me to wean myself, decided to go to Chicago for millinery stock. She invited me to accompany her as far as Milwaukee, where I could select an office if I so desired.

Cousin Ernest met us at the boat with a team of beautiful horses and took us to the Plankinton Hotel, where he lived. After luncheon we went to his office, elegantly furnished and hung with many oil paintings purchased in Europe. We finished the day with sight-seeing.

There had been no mention of my practice until Aunt Julia suggested, "It has been such a full day; hadn't you better wait until tomorrow to look at offices?"

I blurted out, "I am going with you to Chicago tonight."

She laughed, "It's a good idea for you to go to Chicago—you've never been there."

In Chicago at five o'clock the next morning, we walked up Water Street, busy at that early hour with its wholesale food markets. I stopped, took a look around, and announced to Aunt Julia, "I like the way it smells here. I shall practice here."

She scorned the idea. "Why, this is just a wholesale street; you know nothing yet about Chicago; you had better choose Milwaukee, where Cousin Ernest could do so much for you. Think of it! You don't have even one acquaintance in Chicago."

Walking to Congress Street, we took the elevated as far as Forty-third Street, and climbed to a third-floor apartment. There Aunt Julia left me while she went back downtown to buy goods.

On her return I informed her, "I have rented the landlady's hall bedroom, with the privilege of using the sitting room as waiting room if I ever have two patients at one time."

My office-bedroom furnishings consisted of a washbowl and slop bucket kept in the closet; a box couch—my Procrustean bed—six inches too short; a Morris chair that could be converted into an examining table by using two large pillows on the seat (Mother's geese furnished the pillows); a bookcase, with a curtain that covered my books on one side, and my instruments and medicines on the other; and a couple of chairs.

I was to pay thirty dollars a month for my room and board, and as I had saved three hundred dollars to begin my practice, I would have ten months to get on my feet.

I returned to the farm, packed up my meager possessions, and made a couple of dresses. When questioned, "Why didn't you go to Milwaukee?" I mystified my listeners by explaining, "I did not see light until we reached Chicago. It was all the colors of the rainbow."

Although I located in Chicago without rhyme or reason, I

never reconsidered or changed my mind, and never at any time have I regretted it. As an ovum, when a single spermatozoon penetrates it, is closed to the entrance of all others, so my mind when Chicago entered it, was no longer open to St. Louis, Boston, Detroit, Milwaukee or any other town. Chicago impregnated me with its future possibilities. Chicago was not my decision. Chicago was my unescapable affinity. If I had ever felt for any man what I had experienced for Chicago—I would not only have proposed and bought both the engagement and wedding rings, but even procured the marriage license.

In Illinois, in 1892, before the day of State Board Examinations, it was necessary to get three recognized physicians to sign an application for a state license to practice. I knew no Chicago physician, but had read of a Dr. Hickey Carr who had received an appointment as intern to Cook County Hospital. I called on her and found a handsome Scotch-Irish woman with a positive personality, who was inclined to be sympathetic and helpful to a young woman physician. She signed my application blank for licensure, and suggested that for the other two signatures I call on Dr. Marie Mergler, Professor of Gynecology in the Northwestern University Woman's Medical School, and Dr. Sarah Hackett Stevenson, Professor of Obstetrics in the same school.

Dr. Mergler received me with great dignity, but when I explained my errand, she inquired, "Do you intend practicing in Chicago?"

She would have thought so had she seen the over-sized sign that was being made to fill the window of my room on the third floor, and another, to swing from the corner of the drug store on Calumet Avenue and Forty-third Street.

She continued, "When young physicians come to me, I try to discourage their practicing in Chicago, for after failing in the big city, they try the small towns, and with little of either funds or courage, fail there too."

I thought of my poor little three-hundred-dollar bank account and my humble hall bedroom, but I was determined not to be balked, and I insisted, "I have made up my mind to use all my money first, then borrow as much as possible, and finally, starve as long as I can before I allow myself to become discouraged."

She looked at me in unconcealed astonishment. "Oh, well, of course, if you have enough money to get on for five years, at the end of that time you will be all right."

I never forgot this interview, for it remained with me like the words of a Delphian oracle, to check or cheer as occasion demanded. When I thought of taking a streetcar to go downtown or return to my office after a call (I always took a streetcar to make the call), I walked and saved my nickels. Many days I had to keep off my feet to let the blisters heal.

After getting Dr. Mergler's signature, I went with some trepidation for Dr. Stevenson's, explaining my errand to her in a most humble, even apologetic way, for she fairly dazzled me with her beauty and aristocratic personality.

However, to my surprise, she immediately took up her pen, and began writing. "So you are going to practice in Chicago? Fine! There is plenty of room for everybody in this big city." And with a bewitching smile and all the courtesy of the great lady that she was, she saw me to the door.

With a license to practice in my possession, I put my foot firmly on the gas. The go-sign was up, and I passed from civilian into professional life. My shingle, painted on both sides and attached like a tail to the string of other doctors' signs at the corner drugstore, swung to and fro. The Chicago wind, simulating the tambourine-beating Salvation Army lassie, rattled and shook it in an apparent effort to direct the attention of the passing public to the new lady doctor who was prepared to treat any ailment from dandruff to bunions.

My ambition was to be as good a doctor as the best man, but I had not the slightest intention of competing with the masculine portion of the profession. I do not know where I got the idea, but I was obsessed with the notion that the world was full of unmarried women who were suffering—perhaps dying—because they could not force themselves to submit to an examination from a male physician. I looked forward to caring for these modest maids, and was sure I would find no time for other patients.

In less than a week of waiting for patients, and before I had had time for worry, I received a telephone call to come at once to the second apartment of the building at Thirty-sixth and Cottage Grove Avenue. I had no telephone, but considered myself lucky that the druggist would deliver messages at any time, day or night. As there was no inkling of the kind of case it might be, I prepared for any emergency and took a streetcar.

I was surprised when I found myself at the home of Dr. Hickey Carr, who ushered me in and began catechizing, "Did you get a call to come at once?"

"Yes," I assented.

"And were you greatly excited? Have you been going over in your mind how you would treat this emergency, that acute disease? Did it give you a great thrill?"

"Yes, it did," I confessed.

"Well, although it is true that there is no one ill, I could not resist the temptation to give you that big thrill. However, I am not so heartless as to get you here and have nothing to offer you. I have an appointment for you to serve three days as emergency physician at the dedication of the Columbian World's Fair. You will be paid ten dollars a day, and have an opportunity to look around the Fair. The appointment came to me, but on account of my approaching confinement, I thought I had better get a substitute. I hated to discriminate among my many doctor friends, and so selected you. When I mentioned your name to Dr. Allport, he said he had known you as a student in Ann Arbor and was really pleased to accept you."

When I announced my World's Fair appointment at the boardinghouse dinner that night, I was looked upon as a real personage. No one could understand how I could get such an appointment so soon after coming to Chicago, with no friends here. Since my expenses were only thirty dollars a month, this appointment shortened that five-year plan to which Dr. Mergler had consigned me, to four years and eleven months.

My first genuine sick call was from a German woman who had

lost two children from so-called "cholera infantum," and now her year-old baby was ill of the same disease. I examined the child and found an acute intestinal infection. At a neighboring drug store I bought a catheter and funnel, with which I irrigated the baby's bowel, and taught the mother to do it. I expressly stated, "Give the baby no food except boiled water, with perhaps a drop of kimmel in it. I will return this evening."

At lunch a fellow boarder, a young Eastern doctor with fine offices, congratulated me. "I hear you had a new patient."

"Yes," and I went on to tell him what I had found and what I had done for the baby.

"Oh dear, oh dear," he exclaimed. "How I wish I could have seen you to tell you that you cannot carry out on such patients all this hospital treatment you have learned. "Why, she undoubtedly has already thrown out the catheter, and called in a doctor who will give the baby some medicine. You must always give medicine to that type of patient, even if no more than sugar or bread pills. And never tell them not to feed a baby. Too bad!"

I went to my little hall-bedroom office, sat down and had a good cry, then and there resolving to give up the practice of medicine and go back to teaching anatomy. If one practiced medicine just to bamboozle the public, I would have none of it. The teaching of anatomy was honest and honorable, and I felt I had been foolish to start into a high-class swindling game.

I had promised to call on the patient that evening, and although I expected to see someone peep through a crack in the curtain without answering the knock at all, I resolutely applied my knuckles to the door. It flew open as if by magic. The sick baby's mother (she weighed about two-hundred pounds) opened her arms, and literally folded me into them, covering my face and neck with kisses. "Er ist besser! Er ist besser!" she fairly shouted.

Feeling that I had a chance to improve my management of the case, I reassured her, "Now if you feel he should have something to eat—"

111

"No! No!" she cried. "I no care if he never eat, if he get well."

She picked up the catheter and funnel with tender, loving hands, and reported, "I wash him so nice, just like you show me."

In her joy, when the baby was well, she took him in her arms, and went from one to another of her neighbors, saying, "If your baby get sick, don't send for them mens doctors. You get the lady doctor. She give you no medicine. She just tell you what to do, and she wash 'em out so nice."

From that day the solution of the problem of a clientele (so difficult for many young physicians) was assured, with little effort on my part. In a short space of time, like spring, it almost burst upon me.

Yet, my big worry was what to charge patients: if too little, I feared that I would run the risk of not properly evaluating my services and of losing the respect of the patient; if too much, I might discourage her. I am always having financial chills regarding doctors' fees.

Early in my first year of practice a woman in the neighborhood came for special treatments. Her first question was, "What do you charge?"

I groaned in spirit. In my dilemma I sought for neutral ground and spoke as nonchalantly as my intense interest would allow, "Oh, the usual fee."

Smiling knowingly, she acquiesced, "That's good. I can pay two dollars all right."

After coming several times and paying each time, she acknowledged, "I very nearly canceled my appointment today because I didn't have the money."

I assured her, "When you owe me, I feel I have money in the bank—and anyway, the important thing is for you to get well."

After many treatments I pronounced, "You're all right."

"That's fortunate," she said, "for I am obliged to leave the city. Am I right in thinking I owe you sixty dollars?"

I nodded, "Correct!" although actually I had never kept track of the amount.

She paid me sixty dollars, and we parted after an affectionate farewell. The next morning at breakfast my landlady inquired, "How much does she owe you?"

When I shook my head and casually remarked, "Nothing! She paid me in full yesterday," great was her surprise and admiration for my business ability.

"She left in the middle of the night, owing three months' rent, her gas bill and many others," she answered. "In fact, she owes all the business people in the building, except you."

I had to smile—the poor soul had never before had anyone with such childlike trust in her, and this confidence was just too precious to lose.

In my anxiety to succeed I put aside everything that might interfere with my career. I had seen how fond people were of money, what people would do to obtain money, and how even a great career might be crushed under the strain of money. Accordingly, I vowed that money should never keep me from reaching my goal. I never kept a book or sent a bill during the first ten years of my practice, theorizing that patients belong to one of three classes: those whom no one could prevent paying their bills; those who never pay any bills, even under pressure; and those, to which group the vast majority of patients belong, who pay their bills if pleased with the service, and if it is humanly possible.

The wherewithal, too often a nightmare to the medical novice struggling for a foothold, never caused me a moment's anxiety. I did not, like Amy McPherson, string up a clothes line on which grateful patients might pin money as a voluntary contribution for my skill, but every day I picked up enough cash laid on my desk so that I never had to draw on the three hundred dollars I had saved to start my career. Often I was able to add to it.

In all the years of my practice, it mattered not what hour of the night, or how bad the reputation of the locality, fear was never my companion except on one occasion.

I had crossed and recrossed viaducts considered dangerous after dark; I had passed saloons from which drunken men had been hurtled by big burly bartenders, and once a man landed directly across my path so that I had to step over his broken, perhaps dead body; I had waited on a lonely corner for a streetcar at two in the morning, and had seen a man with a bag held up by a thug, who was in hiding behind a pole; I had heard the man with the bag curse the fellow, and order him to get back behind the pole; I had seen the man walk on, leaving me with the robber, who came across the street to my side, where it seemed as if he remained for an hour before shifting to a position behind me, as finally on padded feet, he ran in pursuit of another victim.

I argued that if I always appeared unconcerned, my enemy would conclude that I was in some way protected, or that I had nothing to lose. In spite of this theory I suffered a terrible fright soon after I had begun practice.

About five years before I came to Chicago, Dr. Cronin, a prominent physician, had been lured out on a night call. His dead body was not found for many weeks after his disappearance. The case was widely publicized, especially as the conspirators in his murder were well-known men. The excitement over this famous murder was probably responsible for my behavior when I was wakened by a ring at the door of my basement office suite, where I was sleeping. It was four o'clock one Sunday morning in July.

I looked out of the reception room window, and saw in front of the house a ramshackle buggy which had been a roost for the hens, an emaciated horse, and a boy of about sixteen.

"What do you want?" I called through the open window.

"Tell the doctor to come. The baby's having convulsions."

"Where is the baby?"

"On Forty-ninth and State Street. I've come to take the doctor there."

"All right," I said. "I'll be ready in a minute."

A young medical woman was spending the night with me, and her eyes grew big with horror when I announced, "This is another Cronin case—I feel sure of it."

She implored me not to go.

"Oh, yes," I argued. "If they are after me, I better meet them when I am suspicious, and more able to outwit them. I shall go. However, if I am not back by six o'clock, notify the police."

I stepped with determination towards the buggy. The boy regarded me with alarm and confusion, but made no sign of moving.

"I thought you were in a hurry?" I gave him an accusing look as I climbed in and seated myself in the shabby turnout.

He seated himself beside me and turned the horse in the opposite direction from where he had told me the baby lived.

"Where are you going?" I shouted. He pulled the horse around, and we went rattling down Grand Boulevard.

When we reached State Street at Forty-ninth, he stopped at the intersection, and ordered: "Get out here, walk two houses down, go between them to the back of the lot, where there's a house. Climb up two stairs to the top floor. It's there!"

I walked through the narrow passage to the house in the rear, and climbed the creaking stairs to find a door opening into a kind of service room. I walked through, and without knocking, opened first a door into a living room, and then a door into a kitchen.

Here I saw a man holding a baby that was in violent convulsions, and two women kneeling before a picture of the Virgin Mary. My fear was transformed into action. I took the baby's temperature. It was 107 degrees. I ordered a washtub and two pails, and in the meantime, I stripped the clothing from the body of the burning baby, and placed it in the tub with its head supported by its father's arms. Both of the faucets ran cold water so that while one pail was filling, I poured the cold water from the other pail over the panting baby until the tub was full. Again I took the baby's temperature to find it had dropped to 101 degrees. The baby opened its eyes and whispered, "Papa!"

I took the baby out of the tub and wrapped a blanket around it. Then I began to ask questions: "When did this begin?"

"The baby took sick yesterday," the father related, "and Dr.

115

Van Doozer, our family doctor, was called. He stayed till two o'clock this morning, but after he had gone, the baby got worse, and we sent for him to come back. He will be here any minute."

Without presenting a bill, or making any explanations for my conduct, I left the house, frankly hoping to foster the thought that I had visited the baby as mediator of the Holy Mother. On my way home I stopped to call on Dr. Van Doozer, who lived only a short way from my office. I told him what I had done for his patient, omitting my foolish fears and the behavior of the boy.

I was amazed when Dr. Van Doozer recounted how he had tried all night to get the parents to consent to his giving the baby a cold bath, and I was amused when I thought how helpless those same people had been to prevent me from doing so, or to stem the tide of my recovery from fear. It must have been a recovery, for never since have I lost confidence in the public, or suspected anyone of attempting to injure me.

During the first year of my practice I marched under the banner "Veni, Vidi, Vici," without consciousness that I was soon to come face to face, both in my private practice and in my family life, with the thing that would test my professional strength more than digging up patients, finding money, or making "snap" diagnoses—the thing to which more than fifty years in the practice of medicine has not yet made me immune.

This test that awaited me and for which I was not prepared came to me early in my second year of practice. It was the death of a patient—a surgical case on whom I had operated with the assistance and under the direction of a very able male surgeon. On opening her abdomen I found nothing that looked pathological, but upon the advice of my consultant I removed both ovaries that he pronounced cystic. The hospital where I operated was poorly equipped, and without doubt the patient was infected during the operation. At any rate, on the second post-operative day signs of peritonitis appeared, and for six harrowing days I remained in almost constant attendance until she died.

During those six anxious days I kept relay after relay of

nurses busy administering treatment that I now consider useless: pills of calomel (2 grains with ½ grain of opium) several times a day, hypodermic injections of camphorated oil, turpentine stupes on the abdomen, continuous vaginal douches, and inhalations of ammonia. Keeping up my own morale as well as that of the patient and her relatives taxed me more than direction of the medical care. I became positively ingenious in interpreting symptoms to inspire hope.

Although I had experienced the thrill of birth many times, the shock of death was strange to me. When the end finally came, I realized that I, her physician, and no one else, must write in statistical form the diagnosis and cause of death—a record to stand for all time, a silent witness to the limitations of my profession. It was as though a judge, without a trial, had pronounced sentence upon himself.

The death certificate, however, did not make an end to all further thought of the patient. Night and day, day and night, at meal time, on going to bed, on rising, while at work, even while talking on other subjects, I went over and over the case. What was really the cause of death? There had been no post-mortem examination though I had urged and urged it. Had I been operating on a case that should have been treated medically? Do cystic ovaries need removal? Perhaps I should have called in another physician. Should I have devoted more time to studying and preparing the patient for operation?

Months passed during which there were times when I cried out, begging my ghostly companion to leave me if for only a few moments, imploring for a little respite, but she never left my side. The patient's body had been given to the worms, but her death had been bequeathed without will or testament to me, to be studied, to be regretted, to be rehearsed over and over. Her relatives and friends had grieved and then gone on with their lives. How surprised they would have been if they had known that I, who had seemed so scientifically calm and unemotional, was wearing myself out with the problem of what might have been done to save that human life.

Death was an Achilles thrust that brought to me a keen and poignant sense of failure and overwhelmed me with helplessness. As a child I understood that the old must die and became reconciled to their death. The old die gradually. The eyes, the feet, the hands all slowly lose their functions. Keenness, clearness, exactness become blinking, straining, fumbling, with less and less seeing, less and less hearing, less and less walking, less and less working, as a ship going out to sea gets smaller and smaller, dimmer and dimmer, until it disappears. But a child's death has nothing natural about it. It is a breach of nature.

When I began practicing, I thought I ought to attend every patient who wanted me. One day I was called for a baby, apparently not very ill. I prescribed, and promised a speedy recovery, but within two hours I was called again to find the child unconscious. Again I prescribed, but when I had returned to my office, haunted by the fear that other complications had arisen, I hurried back. The baby had a normal temperature, and to all appearances, was well.

Alice asked me, "Why do you take care of babies?"

"Because I am afraid no one will ever have confidence in me if I refuse to see any patient."

She insisted, "You can never do your best work in such an anxious frame of mind."

Leaning on her approval, I gave up caring for sick babies and turned them over to other doctors.

If the child, however, was a surgical case, I enjoyed operating, and have been fortunate in having lost but two children in many operations.

The mother of one of these children was a Jewess, married many years when she came to me for relief from sterility. After months of treatment we were rewarded, and one day I laid in her arms a beautiful baby girl.

When the child was about five years old, I was called, and only a moment was necessary to diagnose a ruptured appendix. I took the child in my arms, and with the mother, drove to the Woman's Hospital, where I consulted Dr. J. B. Murphy.

He put his hand on the child's abdomen, and said, "Operate at once." I did so, and found a ruptured appendix whose culture showed a streptococcic infection.

In twenty-four hours the child was dead.

I was frenzied with grief. I could not eat or sleep. In my misery I called Dr. Murphy on the telephone, and said, "Dr. Murphy, that child you saw with me died twenty-four hours after the operation. It was a streptococcic ruptured appendix. Do you think if I had—"

With great understanding and still greater sympathy the famous surgeon interrupted me with these words, "My dear girl, I know just how you feel, but you must forget it. That child was doomed before you or I ever saw her. Operate on another patient as soon as you get an opportunity. Don't let this ruin a good surgeon."

Such understanding and kindly advice from a great man brought me back to a courageous and healthy state of mind, and my gratitude has grown with the years.

Two months after I encountered death in my medical practice, it touched my immediate family. I was thirty years of age, and up to that time a doctor had never been called for the sickness of any one of us. I was, therefore, much disturbed when I received a telegram from the farm asking me to come at once on account of the illness of my father. I was especially worried because all the trains out of Chicago were tied up in the big railroad strike of 1894.

I went to the railway station. I must go, train or no train! But how? No one would say when a train might start for Detroit. I boarded a car. I took a seat. I sat in the motionless car all night.

During those long hours of waiting I recalled how Father, while attending the World's Columbian Exposition the previous year, had wanted to give me money, and I had nonchalantly refused it. Alice had told him about my blistering my feet to save carfare. Now I wished more than I could tell that I had accepted help, just to please him. It would have been impossible

119

for Father to understand that I was so much in love with the practice of medicine that even blistering my feet gave me a sense of devotion to a great profession, rather than a feeling of abuse.

Father loved the railroad and I remembered, as I sat in the poorly lighted car, how hard he had worked to have a spur of the Michigan Central from Detroit to Bay City surveyed through Rochester. From one end of the township to the other Father and I had driven, visiting farmers and trying to induce them to contribute money or right of way. I grew warm reliving the excitement of that day in 1876 when the first engine came puffing into Rochester. Father and I had joined the rabble, shrieking a welcome and admiring the big iron horse that would now take our crops to Detroit instead of Father, who always spent two days and nights hauling them with horses and wagons over poor corduroy roads.

The sharp whistle of an engine recalled those days when Father used to drive me back and forth to school. From the top of the hill leading into Rochester the railroad track could be seen for a long distance. If a train was approaching, he would stop the horses and watch the lumbering, lurching freight cars as they moved slowly under a streamer of thick black smoke until the little red caboose was out of sight. Then, chirruping to the horse and slapping her back with the reins, he would remark, "God didn't make that. Man made it. Isn't it beautiful?"

A sudden jolt of the car brought me back from those days that seemed so long ago, to my present anxiety. It was morning and the train was moving. I was on my way.

When I arrived at the farm, I found that Father had had a severe headache several days before, and that since then, his gait had been peculiar. After a few steps he began to walk more and more rapidly until, to reach his destination, he would break into a run. In order to have specialists and hospital care I took him on the train to Harper Hospital in Detroit. He was admitted as a patient of Dr. J. H. Carstens (my old friend of the Woman's Hospital). Dr. Carstens did not shy from examining him and then calling in several neurologists, "who," he said, "will know no more than I do and, I fear, can do nothing for him."

As he had predicted, no one could help my father, and after lying in a semi-comatose condition for two weeks, he died.

A post-mortem examination, upon which I insisted, although it was not a routine procedure, revealed no cause for death. I accompanied the body back to the farm. It was July and intensely hot. The undertaker who took charge of Father's body asked me to apply cloths moistened in a disinfectant solution every two hours. In spite of this care it became necessary before the day set for the funeral to close the casket, but not before I had seen my father's body slowly disintegrate into a loathsome mass of corruption.

The loss of my father left me with a sense of loneliness. Hunger for his approval nagged me year after year. As a doctor I had kept a professional vigil at his bedside for those two anxious weeks before he died, had shouldered the abhorrent task of caring for the corpse, but I had had no twinges of conscience, no self-depreciation.

On the other hand, the loss of a patient starts me to question and forbids reconciliation. It develops in me an inferiority complex mingled with guilt. Standing by the post-mortem table and facing the pathological cause of death, I am overpowered by my own inefficiency and the helplessness of my profession.

I once heard Dr. Charles Mayo say that the path of progress was lined with tombstones, and I am sure that every death is for some doctors the impetus for a prolonged and thorough study of the case. At the present time, in many of our cities, physicians meet and study the causes of all of the important and puzzling deaths that have occurred during the week.

It has taken many years and much suffering for me to learn that to die is as natural as to be born; that without death birth would become a greater tragedy than death could ever be.

DR. WILL MAYO

WHEN I first visited the Mayo Clinic, I was fascinated with the simple technique of Dr. William Mayo. He was so sure of himself that you felt sure of him. During the operation you were with him, not at a distance, but close by. You grew under his tuition as plants grow in the sun, but though you became inspired to become something bigger and better, you never found in a Mayo clinic any food for your ego. When you arrived, you may have been conscious of some degree of superiority, but when you departed, that bubble had burst, and with bowed head you dedicated yourself to hard work, persistent study, renewed honesty to self, and loyalty to scientific endeavor.

I was present when a young physician visiting the Clinic remarked in a stage whisper as Dr. Will was putting the last sutures in the incision, "Did you notice that Dr. Mayo left a sponge in the abdomen?"

Dr. Mayo glanced at the speaker, and carelessly replied, "You couldn't have been paying close attention. I always leave in two sponges, to keep the bowels warm."

The visiting doctors bantered the smart guy so unmercifully that he left town that night, and Dr. Mayo's remark was, "I envied him. He had just finished his internship, and will never again know as much as he does today."

12

A WOMAN SURGEON'S ARMAGEDDON

NO PROFESSION demands more attention to detail, or consumes more time than medicine. Every day I made new acquaintances, patients, with whom I became intensely intimate. Every day I solved so many knotty problems that were vexing people that my pleasure in them was an anesthetic for my own difficulties and discomforts.

Unused to city transportation, I enjoyed riding in horse-drawn or cable streetcars, and when I climbed the long flight of stairs to ride on the elevated, I experienced the thrill that an airplane gives youngsters today. Since I was a total stranger to Chicago, I enjoyed learning the names of the streets, public buildings and parks. Even the alleys held interest for me. because many of my patients lived in homes that were located on them.

In my second year of practice I often had so many calls that I rented a horse from the neighboring livery stable. One day, when my practice had reached the point where I had rented the horse every day for a week, the manager of the stable came to me. "I think you need a horse and ought to buy one."

"I haven't enough money and will not go in debt."

"How much could you pay?"

"Only seventy-five dollars."

"You may have the horse for that, and I will throw in the harness, buggy—yes, the whip and the lap robe."

How proud I was to be a real horse-and-buggy doctor at last! When I told one of my loyal German patients of my luck, she insisted that I needed her dog to watch the horse and buggy while I made calls, and she gave him to me.

He was a mongrel, part fox and part bull terrier, a devoted and intelligent animal. Fritz slept on the foot of my bed, and whenever I started out with the horse and buggy, took his place just at the back of Kit's heels, and kept up with her no matter how far or how fast she traveled.

When I would get out of the buggy, Fritz would jump in, taking his seat with the importance of a king opening parliament. But if any children came around, out jumped Frittie, and woe to the child who did not beat a retreat! He barked so loudly and savagely that his whole body shook, nor did he hesitate to grasp the leg of a person caught meddling with the horse or buggy.

Occasionally, after long trips, I missed him, but when I returned to the house, he was there to welcome me, or soon appeared. I looked at his wagging tail and wriggling body, and wondered how he had been able to find his way back in a city, over strange roads.

He was devoted to calling on the sick. One day Ray, the colored man who cared for the horses, held him in his arms until I had left the house. When the dog heard the retreating hoofs of the horse, he sprang from Ray's arms, and dashed through the office to the front doorway. It was closed with a locked screen, but bolts and bars offered no impediment, for he burst through the center of the wire screen, and in a few seconds was ambling behind Kit's hind feet.

Kit often became tired of too long a wait and would set out for home, dragging the hitching weight along with her. Fritz, however, would never desert her or the buggy, and when a policeman would try to take Kit and Fritz, like lost children, to the nearest police station, it was no easy job, for Fritz became so savage that it took a number of policemen to get them to the station. When I found both horse and dog gone, I called up the police and invariably found them waiting for me, and the police glad to get rid of Frittie.

Up to the time that I came to Chicago I had always held jobs that engaged every minute of my time. Consequently, I could not reconcile myself to a Micawber period of waiting, and fearing to parallel Dr. McLean's first year in St. Louis, with its pitiful scarcity of patients—none, in fact—it occurred to me to look for an opportunity to teach anatomy.

I waited only for my license before I applied to the Northwestern University Woman's Medical School for an instructorship in anatomy, and got it. There was no salary attached to this apparently unpopular position, but I was so eager for work that I might have been willing to pay for it if I had had money. After finding a transportation that would cost only ten cents a day, I devoted every afternoon during my first year of practice to dissecting and prosecting.

Although demonstrating anatomy every afternoon often tore my practice schedule to pieces, it gave me an opportunity to associate with women doctors. Many of them were full professors, held hospital positions, and conducted clinics. I especially prized teaching women medical students, and when, at the end of the year, a group of students asked permission to take a summer course under me privately and recompense me for it, I felt well repaid for the year's work.

When they requested credit for the proposed course, the reply of the professor of anatomy amazed them. He told them, "If you choose to have my nephew, who is an excellent demonstrator of anatomy and a very good teacher, I will see that you have credit, but any money paid for a summer course must go to him."

The incensed girls did not take the summer course, but in the fall I received notice that my services were no longer needed. In my pique, I wept.

Dogged, and determined to keep my connection with the Woman's Medical School, I applied to Dr. Sarah Hackett Stevenson, Professor of Obstetrics, for a chance to teach in her department. She met me with gracious enthusiasm.

"Yes," she said, "I am very anxious to put in a course of embryology. I should like to have you teach it."

I told her frankly, "When I graduated, the University of Michigan did not give us a course in embryology, and I am not familiar with the subject, but I will begin studying at once and be ready to teach next year."

She smiled sweetly, but her answer was firm. "You will give it now or never."

I had a vivid recollection of my worry and self-depreciation when, unprepared, I had taught calisthenics in St. Louis. I shall never forget my feverish haste to acquire enough knowledge to keep a two-weeks' jump ahead of the classes. I sweated at the thought of those long hot days in midsummer when I dissected every day, from four in the morning until noon, to prepare myself to demonstrate anatomy in the fall. Yet what I had done twice I ought to be able to do a third time. I did not hesitate. My reply was as firm as hers had been. "Now."

So it came to pass that for the third time I tackled a job for which I was wholly unprepared. To add to the tragi-comic situation, the college possessed no incubator, demonstrating material, or appropriation with which to purchase any apparatus.

Lady Luck must have loved me when she led me to the late Dr. Frank Wynekoop, Professor of Embryology in the College of Physicians and Surgeons (University of Illinois College of Medicine), who offered not only to teach me, but to incubate the eggs for class demonstration. For more than a year he generously gave me every Sunday and so many evenings that the students never discovered what a cuckoo I was, laying my eggs in another's nest.

One of my students, Alice Lindsay, a charming titian-haired beauty, took upon herself the burdensome duty of carrying the eggs back and forth from the college. The egg trips hatched into a romance and Dr. Wynekoop married Alice five years after her graduation.

arm and with the tip of one finger lightly touched his wrist.

"What are you made of?" he exclaimed and sat up on the table.

I tried to arch my eyebrows *a la* Mother and give her laugh of finality. It must have had an effect, for he left the room and ever after treated me with the utmost courtesy.

Clinics demand hospital service, without which many patients cannot be cared for. For this reason the staff of the Columbia Dispensary opened a hospital in the ghetto near the clinic. In the latter part of the nineteenth century laws governing the establishment and conduct of hospitals were so lax that any individual or group could rent a building one week and open an unstandardized hospital the next.

This hospital had such a fleeting existence that it was never named. I was among the first to send in a patient, an operative case—a minor operation that I was able to perform without assistance. The day after the operation I visited the hospital, but could not get in. Every door, front and back, was locked; windows were closed and shades drawn. Determined to see my patient, I looked around for an open window. Discovering one in the basement, I crawled through and fell into a coal bin. Smudged and excited, I climbed the cellar stairs to find the nurses and servants huddled in the dark kitchen.

From them I learned that on the previous day there had been a death in the hospital and the neighbors, en masse and armed with sticks and knives, had threatened the staff and the nurses. Laughing at their fears, I called an ambulance to remove my patient, who was in good condition, to another institution and left the hospital by the front door. This was my first and worst hospital experience in Chicago.

The hospital as well as the Columbia dispensary closed; and another hospital and dispensary with the same staff opened at Twenty-fourth and Dearborn Streets. It was called the Charity Hospital and here Dr. Robinson gave me both a gynecological clinic and the opportunity to operate on every third patient referred from my clinic to the hospital.

This move brought the clinic within a short distance from my

My acquaintance with Drs. Frank and Alice Lindsay Wynekoop was the beginning of a lifelong friendship—a prelude to a love that grew even after the tragedy which engulfed Alice—the murder of Rheta Wynekoop, of which she was to be accused years later.

I had never conducted or even attended a dispensary clinic during my medical-school days or in the four years of residencies, except a weekly private clinic in the New England Hospital.

Nevertheless, my connection with the Woman's Medical School was making me aware that a dispensary clinic was a wonderful method for continuous post-graduate study.

One day on the way to the college where I was teaching, I met by chance one of my Ann Arbor classmates who suggested my going to Dr. Byron Robinson for some clinical work. I acted at once and obtained a gynecological and obstetrical dispensary clinic at the Columbia Dispensary, located in the heart of the ghetto.

With an opportunity to teach and build up a new department in Northwestern University Woman's Medical School and the chance to work independently in a clinic with Dr. Robinson, I was rich beyond my fondest, even wildest expectations.

As my clinical hours were from eight to ten in the morning, I was always on duty an hour before any other member of the staff showed up. I had been holding the clinic about a month when, one morning, I arrived and found that a short, dapper young physician was already there. He walked into my room without rapping, locked the door and put the key into his pocket. Sprawling across the table like a frog for dissection, he called out, "I have a fever! Feel my head!"

I was scrubbing my hands and lifted them in mute recognition of his presence.

"Feel my pulse! Feel my pulse!" he panted.

I was standing in front of the mirror and my imagination reflected in it the old bay mare moving slowly from side to side in the pasture lot to avoid the advances of the jumping stallion.

Keeping as far as possible from the table, I stretched out my home, but cut out the obstetrical service, in which I was wholeheartedly interested. I loved obstetrics, but at the same time I was keenly aware of its unpopularity. I understood perfectly the bitter resentment of Dr. Joseph B. DeLee, the greatest of our modern obstetricians, when he wrote in the preface of his huge text book: "The present notorious disapprobation and disesteem of obstetrics . . . ."

Because I was a woman, to specialize in obstetrics would brand me as a midwife, a Cinderella step-sister of the usurping "man-midwife". Perhaps in the long run it might be wiser to apply myself to surgery until I had gained recognition as a surgeon—then I could turn my attention to obstetrics. Entering obstetrics through a surgical door, I could work in the birthroom with skill and distinction. For such reasons I hoped to become an independent surgeon.

Anatomy, to which I had devoted much time, is the best foundation upon which to build any specialty. My four-years' hospital experience would serve as a scaffold by which to climb to higher levels, and now constructive instruction in operative surgery by Dr. Byron Robinson, whose assistant I was, would provide a blueprint for a surgical specialty.

Dr. Robinson, a pedagogic prodigy, was in addition, a man of abstemious habits and devoted to the study of anatomy and surgery; but in his personal appearance and language, unpolished and homely. He never euphemized, but always used the word "gut" instead of "intestine," and the word "belly" instead of "abdomen."

Whenever the rectum is dilated, the anesthetized patient will take a deep breath that sounds very much like the heehaw of a donkey. At such a demonstration, Dr. Robinson always made the remark, "Hear the braying of the ass."

His listeners attributed to him a coarse and vulgar mind, but I, fortunately, being country-bred like Dr. Robinson, understood him. This homespun vernacularism did not prevent his being the cleanest of men mentally and morally, honest as a Dutchman, unprejudiced towards sex or social ranking, and indefatigable as a worker and teacher. With his students he was ruthless. Only he who wished to be instructed and helped was able to endure the wounds given his pride.

I had worked with Dr. Robinson for two very happy and profitable years, when one day I read the description of an operation by Dr. Howard Kelly, of Baltimore. The next day, without consulting Dr. Robinson, I had started an operation and was proceeding to carry out the Kelly technique when Dr. Robinson inquired, "What are you doing?"

I explained, "I am performing the Kelly operation."

At that, he dropped the instrument he was holding, turned quickly, and left the room.

Nothing remained but to finish the operation with the assistance of the intern and nurse in an atmosphere of silence that rivaled the grave.

I thought too much of Dr. Robinson, and was too grateful to him not to hasten to talk the matter over to an understanding. I found that in a gynecological meeting the previous evening he had denounced this particular operation of Dr. Kelly's, and I could hardly blame him when he insisted that henceforth I must talk over with him every operation that I did.

With tears and sobs I begged his pardon and acquiesced to all his requests. Nevertheless, I began at that moment to realize that I must become an independent operator. Why shouldn't I? I had to stand alone when unsuccessful. Hence, if I stood alone at all times, I would enjoy and get the credit for success.

He had often said in my presence that it was worth while to train Van Hoosen because she knew her anatomy. Dr. Robinson himself never discontinued his dissecting. Late into the night he could be found carefully dissecting the sympathetic system or the circulation of the uterus. In my teaching, while instructor in anatomy in the University of Michigan Medical School for two years, as well as in the Northwestern University Women's Medical School for another year, I had handled and been responsible for the dissecting of over a hundred bodies. Dr. Robinson almost envied me my anatomical knowledge, and certainly took great pleasure and pride in teaching me, though often he criticized to the point of abuse.

"How can you stand such treatment?" the visiting doctors would ask.

I would reply, "When I have learned to use the knife, the wounds to my pride and sensibilities will soon heal."

Relying upon the splendid training that I had received in the New England Hospital for Women and Children in Boston, and the two years' association with Dr. Byron Robinson in Chicago, I took steps to acquire independence in operating. Dr. Rachel Hickey Carr agreed to help me in any operation I wished to do. To find a hospital that would allow a young would-be surgeon to operate is difficult even today. Fortunately, on the South Side near my home was a hospital whose superintendent was a woman physician. Here, with no difficulty I obtained permission to operate. My first patient was a Jewess who needed a corrective gynecological operation. I had been well-trained in the technique of this operation, which involved no risk to life and should be very successful. Nevertheless, soon after the operation the patient had a rise of temperature and before the end of a week every stitch hole, as well as the incision, was spouting pus. There was yellow pus, green pus, thick pus, and thin pus. The wound gaped widely open. Week after week passed, and still the purulent wound did not close.

It was nearly two months before that patient was in condition to leave the hospital, and it was not surprising that her husband refused to pay the very large bill. The superintendent told him that he could not remove his wife until he had paid the hospital. "Very well," the man bluffed, "you keep my wife." Finally I prevailed upon him to pay the hospital instead of me.

This case had taught me so much that I didn't feel like a martyr, nor did I feel that I had been robbed. During the weeks that I had dressed the wound I discovered that the nurses did not understand how to sterilize sponges, or properly prepare the operating room. Quite by accident one day I found the nurses wearing sterile gowns and gloves, but making sponges from a roll of gauze just as it had come from the factory. This gauze had been marked "sterile gauze," but they did not seem to understand that this label meant nothing, and that sponges should be freshly sterilized before an operation. This easily accounted for the deluge of pus that very nearly drowned my ambitions, not to mention the patient and her purse.

For the next operation that I performed in that hospital I did all the sterilizing in my own small laboratory at home. I purchased cheap containers called "telescopes," large enough to hold gowns, sheets, sponges, etc., and a fish kettle for instruments. Everything that was to be used in the operating room I sterilized, packed, and took in the buggy with me to the hospital. I left instructions to make no preparations other than to have the operating room clean. Long before the time set for the operation, I arrived, wiped all the furniture with lysol solution, unpacked and set up the operating room. We allowed no nurse in the room. I took charge of the instruments and Dr. Carr, the sponges. In this laborious manner, month on month, we did all manner of operations. We never had another case of infection, and as we troubled no one, we were exceedingly popular with everyone at the hospital.

So far all the teaching or clinical appointments in the field of medicine where I was trying to embed my embryonic future had come to me more by accident than through any recognition of my fitness or achievements: emergency physician in the Columbian Exposition, demonstrator of anatomy in the Northwestern University Woman's Medical School, Professor of Embryology in the same school, clinical assistant in gynecology in the Columbia, and later in the Charity Hospital and dispensary, obstetrician in the outpatient department of the Columbia dispensary. Last, but not least, I was an independent surgeon.

Taking into consideration that, in my hotheaded infatuation for Chicago, I had begun practicing in a city where I had not a single friend or acquaintance, I should have been satisfied with my luck, but I was not.

My ambition was to have the position seek me, and I was gratified when the late Dr. I. N. Danforth summoned me to his office to ask if I would consider taking the position of Professor of Obstetrics in the Northwestern University Women's Medical School if a vacancy should occur. Without waiting for this event, in two weeks he again invited me to meet him and offered me a gynecological service on the staff of the Wesley Hospital.

This was my first worth-while position. It put me in close association with one of Chicago's ablest gynecologists, Dr. Thomas Watkins. He was a wonderful man—kind, tolerant, fair and the sweetest character I ever knew. Beloved by all, he had no enemies.

This gynecological service was divided between us, six months for each. A week before his service ended, he would turn over to me all the operative cases, saying, "As long as you will have the post-operative care of these patients you better operate on them."

One delightful picture of Dr. Watkins and his contemporary, the distinguished psychologist Dr. Daniel Brower, remains very vivid. One day, fearful of the proverbial large family of the clergy, a forty-five-year-old bride of a Methodist minister entered my service asking for a hysterectomy. I refused on the ground that there was no indication for such an operation. When Dr. Watkins took the service, she returned and renewed her request. Finding that I had sent her away, Dr. Watkins called Dr. Brower and me in consultation.

I stood on one side of the bed and Dr. Watkins on the other, each holding one of the patient's hands, while Dr. Brower examined her. On finishing, he stepped to the foot of the bed, and with both hands raised, he pronounced his ultimatum. "Madam, do not be impatient. The Lord is performing a hysterectomy on you, and such a hysterectomy as Watkins never dreamed of." Dr. Watkins' face was a study.

Two years saw the end of my service in the Wesley Hospital, which closed for the erection of a new building.

The loss of this delightful hospital service was through no fault of mine and was more keenly mourned because it was followed almost immediately by my breaking connections with the Charity Hospital. In this, too, I had no share in the blame.

Dr. Franklin Martin, a fine surgeon and wonderful organizer, was Chief of Staff of the hospital. He was the antithesis of Dr. Robinson and it was only a matter of time for these two strong characters to become set against each other. I was never interested in the exact cause of the clash, but when Dr. Robinson was expelled, I, like the placenta of the newborn, was included in the expulsion.

Treating as many as seventy patients in an afternoon at the Charity dispensary, operating almost every day at the Wesley Hospital, together with teaching embryology had occupied every minute of my time. To be suddenly deprived of all this work except the teaching was naturally depressing, but I did not have long to cry.

Almost immediately following these losses I was urged to organize and give first-aid courses in the Home Economics Department of Armour Institute. These courses were well paid for, and took less time than the hospital work.

After fifteen years of teaching first aid in the Armour Institute and ten years in the Lewis Institute, lack of time forced me to retire in favor of another woman physician.

In 1896 one of Chicago's leading surgeons, the first woman doctor in the world to perform independent surgery, died. Her body lay in state in the Women and Children's Hospital that she had founded in 1865—the first nonsectarian hospital in Chicago and one of the four hospitals in the United States having a staff composed entirely of women physicians. Long lines of weeping mourners streamed through the hospital doors to look upon the familiar face of beautiful, motherly Dr. Mary Harris Thompson.

The vacancy left by the death of Dr. Thompson opened up to the medical woman who could fill it an opportunity of a lifetime. This position, Chief of Staff, was by far the best hospital opening in the Middle West. That I did not at once accept when approached by the trustees, and go to any lengths to fill the place is unbelievable.

My only reason for turning down such an offer was that I feared it would take so much of my time that I could not meet my obligations. I was the sole breadwinner in the family; Sarah, my niece, was not well; and, besides a $10,000 life insurance policy, I had assumed the burden of a heavy mortgage.

I was very happy when I learned that Dr. Lucy Waite, the wife of Dr. Byron Robinson, had been appointed to the position. Shortly after her appointment she asked me to take charge of the obstetrical department. I consented providing I might be released if the services interfered too much with my practice.

In a very short time I was enamored of the position. I found chances for research and improvement in clinical methods. The post-partum patients were getting three vaginal douches a day and when I stopped them the annoying temperatures disappeared. Many patients who came for delivery had old severe lacerations of the perineum. Immediately, or on the day following delivery, I repaired these old tears, and discharged the patients in excellent condition. To my great surprise, many patients who were turned over to me paid good fees.

After a year of delightful service I learned that plans for setting up a school of midwifery were on foot. My belligerency towards such a project was no secret and was given as the reason for my resignation that I sent to the trustees.

At the very end of the nineteenth century, on the advice of my dear friend, Dr. Rachael Hickey Carr, I became a staff member of the Provident Hospital, an institution for the training of colored nurses. Besides the superintendent, a few of the trustees and the staff were white. The patients were both white and negro.

My interest in race problems made my appointment a very natural happening. Although I had never seen a negro until I went to college, my country training and early life had made me free from prejudices and had produced in me a condition that I call "color blindness to races". I once inadvertently demonstrated this blindness by kissing one of my most beautiful and lovable colored patients. If I had struck her in the face she could not have been more surprised or shocked. I never repeated my blunder.

In this hospital I learned the value and pleasure of gracious manners. I am convinced that the colored people are the only group in the United States that, under all circumstances, are kind and polite by nature.

I remained more or less actively connected with the staff until the hospital was moved to the building previously used by the Chicago Lying In Hospital.

Out of the hundreds of white patients that I operated on at this hospital, not one ever complained or was dissatisfied. In fact, each patient recommended the hospital to others, and in this way made it easy for me to send my patients to a hospital for colored people. The service in this small hospital was better than in many larger institutions.

Many lifelong and worth-while friends, both colored and white, became mine through this connection, but my friendship with Alf Anderson was the one on which I set most value. He had a massive head, like the model of a great master, balanced on a body so warped and twisted that, even with the help of crutches, he could hardly walk. It was with difficulty that he ate his meals.

He was the hospital bookkeeper when I first knew him, filling his spare time composing songs (he wrote one for Melba) and operas. Later he became the editor of *The Defender,* and during the last years of his short life he financed and conducted a lovely summer resort about sixty miles south of Chicago, where his people could have privileges which were denied them elsewhere.

When my spirits were low, I used to visit the Providence Hospital at six o'clock in the morning, in time for the nurses' devotional hour. In a beautiful green room, furnished only by a very large chair and a grand piano, I sat and watched those trim, young colored girls kneel and sing, sing and kneel, in an inspiring Episcopalian service. Then I took breakfast with them, usually chatting afterward for an hour with Alf Anderson.

When I left the hospital my poor, pale troubles had been blacked out, and I was able to face the day with something akin to the spirit that has animated and supported the colored people through almost a century of unjust discrimination.

One day when I had accidentally learned that the position

of Head of Gynecology and Obstetrics in the University of Michigan Medical School was vacant, I took the night train to Ann Arbor. Arriving at seven in the morning, I went straight to the home of my friend, Dr. Victor C. Vaughn, dean of the medical school. He was glad to see me and asked, "How long are you going to stay in Ann Arbor?"

"I am going to stay until I have received the appointment of Professor of Obstetrics and Gynecology."

The doctor was greatly disconcerted, but I was determined. I had spent money, and more important, time, to come to get the position. We had some long talks on the subject, during which Dr. Vaughn sadly confessed, "You cannot have the appointment, much as I would like to see you get it, because you are a woman."

When I left him to take the evening train back to Chicago, I said, "Goodbye, Doctor. I think it is important, just for the principle of it, that a woman occupy the position of Professor of Gynecology in a coeducational medical school, and I am going back to Chicago to get such a position. If my own university will not adminster justice to my sex, I will find some other school that will."

Not long after, through the death of Dr. Marie Mergler, one of the finest and most able surgeons and teachers in Chicago, a vacancy for Professor and Head of Gynecology on the faculty of the Northwestern University Woman's Medical School occurred. I was appointed to fill this position but after teaching for nine proud and happy months, my professorship that carried with it two hospital appointments, floated away as if it had been a dream. I was eating an early breakfast one March morning, expecting to hold an eight o'clock college clinic, when I happened to glance at the headlines of the Chicago *Daily Tribune:* NORTHWESTERN UNIVERSITY WOMAN'S MEDICAL SCHOOL CLOSED.

It was very definite, and absolutely final. I never knew the reason for this action, or the suddenness of it—two months before the end of the school year. No disposition had been made for students, teachers, or teaching material. As in an earthquake, the earth had opened and the Northwestern University Woman's Medical School had disappeared. I had now no teaching or college position, no clinic, no hospital appointment, but I did have my private practice and my adoring family. Best of all, I was still young and had a fair equipment to find other openings.

About two weeks after this catastrophe, opportunity knocked. I met **Dr. William Quine**, dean of the College of Physicians and Surgeons (University of Illinois College of Medicine). He inquired, "What are you doing since the Woman's Medical School has been closed?"

I bragged, "I am chief gynecologist and surgeon in my own private practice."

"That's fine!" he said. "How would you like to be Professor of Clinical Gynecology in the College of Physicians and Surgeons, and conduct a surgical clinic every week?"

I retorted, "Nothing would please me more!"

He left with, "Come to my office soon; we'll talk it over."

When I called at Dr. Quine's office, he did not keep me waiting. He put before me the requirements for holding a clinical position in a coeducational medical school. "The students are a rough lot. I have known them to put a professor that they did not like right out of the window! Do you realize that to hold a surgical clinic every week, month in and month out, demands recourse to a wealth of surgical material? Can you operate so automatically that you can give at the same time a lecture both systematic and instructive?"

After more than a half hour of talk on the requisites for the position of Professor of Clinical Gynecology and the holding of a regular weekly surgical clinic, he scrutinized me keenly with his sharp blue eyes and challenged, "Can you do all this?"

I did not hesitate. I made no explanation. I raised my fist and brought it down on his desk with a thud that set all the papers rattling and the ink bottle jumping, and swore, "I will!"

He smiled one of his beautiful smiles. "Now, isn't that remarkable? That is the only answer I would have accepted, and I didn't even know it."

At that time, I was not aware that the majority of the faculty were strongly against me on the acknowledged ground of sex, and that it meant a faculty fight, with the odds against the dean.

Dr. Rachelle Yarros, who, as a teacher of obstetrics was a member of the faculty, informed me, "When Dean Quine put your name up for faculty appointment, it met with indifference and was handed over to the executive committee. They, in turn, handed it to the faculty appointment committee, but without recommendation. The faculty appointment committee handed it back, also without recommendation, and so it was passed from one committee to another. I never knew just what was done to put it over, but Dean Quine is very clever. I once heard him say when the faculty had turned down something that he wanted very much, 'All right, gentlemen. Disgrace your dean, if you wish. You have that privilege!' And of course, after such a remark, he had his way."

It was more than a month before I received word of my appointment. One night, near midnight, the telephone rang, and I answered.

The voice said, "Who is this?"

I answered, "Dr. Van Hoosen."

The voice replied, "Oh, no, who is this?"

I again gave my name, but the voice insisted, "Oh, no."

At this I shouted, "Well, who do you think it is?"

It was Dr. Quine boasting, "I am speaking to the Professor of Clinical Gynecology of the College of Physicians and Surgeons! Drop into my office soon. Good night."

I went to his office, where we planned my campaign, for we both knew that there would be a fight. Because only a small class remained for the summer term, I was to begin my clinics in June (my lucky month). The course was to be elective so that any student who was opposed to being taught by a woman would not be obliged to attend. Lastly, the clinics were to be open to junior students only, thus obviating comparisons, since the seniors were taught by the older members of the faculty.

The summer term opened the first of June, allowing only six

weeks for making preparations! I shuddered at how conspicuous I would be, for I saw myself under the spotlight, with its heat almost literally consuming me. What could I do to protect myself? Suddenly, it came to me that if I could present a patient, unusual and rare, unlike any patient the students had ever seen or heard of, it might be possible to shift the spotlight from me to the patient, and I might be spared humiliation in my first encounter with the student body.

I recalled a twenty-six-year-old woman living in North Dakota, who had a very unusual congenital condition known as hypospadia, and exstrophy of the bladder. That is, from her navel, down through the pubis and the external genitals to the rectum, she was open—practically wrong side out. It was possible to look directly into the urinary bladder. The pelvic bones were widely separated, and all the external genital organs split in the manner of a harelip. She had no control of her secretions, and sat all day on a commode chair. I determined to send for her, pay her expenses, put her in the West Side Hospital adjoining the college, keep her there till the day of that first clinic, and then present and demonstrate her abnormality. Later, at another clinic, I would operate.

My poor pitiful patient arrived, and I visited her daily, not only as a doctor, but as a friend, lest she might get homesick and leave. Never did a patient get such assiduous and delicate attention!

The dreaded day came. I went to the college, accompanied by a trusted woman physician who would give the anesthetic. The nurse in charge of the clinical amphitheater and the two young men student assistants, with every move, every look, every monosyllable, insulted me. I was choking with fright, my knees shook like aspens. The patient clung desperately to me, never loosening her grasp on my hand till deeply asleep.

When I extricated myself and walked to the scrubroom, I glanced through the crack between the double doors leading into the amphitheater, and saw the only thing I had not expected or prepared for. There was not a student in the amphitheater! It was a freeze-out! My legs stiffened, my fear vanished. I was enraged! Not to give me even one chance!

I returned to the patient and the two men students, threw off the covering and revealed her rare and terrible affliction. One young man disappeared, and the other was lost in the mystery of congenital pathology. "What is it?" he whispered.

I replied, "Hypospadia, with exstrophy of the bladder." I knew he had never heard the words, and I pronounced them as rapidly as I could.

The other young man soon returned and asked, "Shall I take the patient into the amphitheater?" adding, "There are some boys in there now."

I spoke thoughtfully, "No, I think not, but would they like to see the patient?"

"Yes," he replied.

"Then tell them to come in."

The students trooped in, single-file, and for nearly three hours I demonstrated my patient. The news had traveled from one classroom to another, and not only junior students, but seniors, sophomore, and even freshmen joined the interested procession. Members of the faculty got word of it, and stepped in to see what it was all about. I never again lacked an audience through all the years that I conducted that weekly surgical clinic.

My troubles, however, were far from being at an end, for although the students were interested in my clinic and I never failed to have patients of teaching value and variety, it was with unexplainable trepidation that at the end of the term I gave an examination. According to custom I had sent in my questions, and appointed proctors to enforce order.

I did not know at the time, but found out afterwards, that some of the students were determined not only to escape an examination, but even to prevent any of the other students from taking it. After a few skirmishes during the writing of the questions on the blackboard, the ringleaders involved the whole class in a riot. There was a free-for-all fight, with such destruction of clothing, breaking of furniture, shrieking and howling that the superintendent of the school, unable to make himself heard, telephoned for the dean.

At the news that the dean was on his way, the confusion ceased. The students were a quiet, cowed bunch when Dr. Quine appeared. He minced no words, and in a few minutes he had the names of six of the ringleaders and expelled them from school. The students came to me with apologies and actual tears, and I in turn appealed to Dr. Quine to give them another trial. He removed the ban, but assured them over and over again that his clemency came from my request, and not through his own volition.

The clinic now ran smoothly, and I could see weekly gains in popularity. Towards the end of the last term at school, I arranged to perform a Caesarean section. As there had not been such an operation performed in that amphitheater for six years, none of the students in the school had ever seen one.

In consequence, the amphitheater that accommodated six hundred was full to overflowing, and included many students from other nearby medical schools. My usual routine had been to give a clinical lecture of about ten minutes while scrubbing my hands in the amphitheater, but on this occasion I scrubbed in the preparation room, entered the operating pit with the patient, and took the knife up immediately. I was sure that with the knife in my hand I would be, as always, oblivious to the crowd or to outside disturbance.

After the operation one of the women doctors present inquired, "How could you be so cool, as if no one were there?"

I told her that it was holding the knife that blotted out the crowd.

The Caesarean section was, as usual, the most spectacular, though in reality the simplest of all surgical procedures. I felt, after this successful clinic, that I had reached a high point in vindicating Dr. Quine's loyal support.

From my pinnacle of success I could not see the shadows falling across my path, but in a week I thought my sun had set. On the Saturday following the Caesarean section, immediately after the clinic, I was handed a letter from the secretary of the West Side Hospital staff (there was only a courtesy affiliation between the hospital and the medical school) stating that in the future I would be denied the privilege of having my patients cared for in their hospital.

When translated into the plan of my life this meant that I would have to give up either my professorship in the college or persuade the hospital staff to rescind their action and take me back. Dr. Danforth, when Dean of the Northwestern Woman's Medical School, once admonished me, "Do not let the grass grow under your feet." I went at once to the president of the hospital staff and from him to each member of the executive board with conciliation—not recrimination. All of them received me with the utmost courtesy, and such consideration that I judged the affair closed.

Shortly after this episode the State Medical Society of Illinois held its annual meeting in Chicago. I was scheduled for a clinic in the amphitheater where I had recently performed the Caesarean operation. This amphitheater was connected with the West Side Hospital, that faces on a street a block away, by means of a passageway over the alley.

For this State Medical Society clinic I arranged to operate on a patient suffering from a severe falling of the womb, that required an operation with a complicated technique of five stages. Not to be disappointed in getting hospital reservations, I went to the president of the West Side Hospital staff and insisted that he give me a note admitting my patient to the ward. He contended that it was not necessary, but finally gave it to me.

I was now confident that no trouble could arise. Nevertheless, on the day for the clinic, I was in the amphitheater one hour before time. After looking over the instruments and arranging the tables in the pit, I asked Dr. Susanne Orton, the anesthetist, to go for the patient.

In a few minutes she returned with the news that the door of the passageway leading from the hospital to the college was locked, and no one knew where the key was.

I surmised a ruse to prevent my holding a clinic, and to checkmate, I said to Dr. Orton, "Go to the hospital, dress the patient quickly, and bring her around by the street to the college. As soon as you have brought her over, anesthetize her, and then wheel her into the amphitheater. I will be waiting to begin the operation. You will have to work fast, for it's now only a few minutes before time to start the clinic, and the seats in the amphitheater are already well filled."

When I entered the pit, the patient was not yet in evidence, but I had unlimited faith in my anesthetist, who was a very direct person and yet, had a reserve that often made her approach rather forbidding.

She afterward related, "I went to the nurse in the hospital, and demanded the patient's clothing. I directed the patient, 'Get dressed at once and come with me.' In silence the patient was dressed, and with locked arms we went from the hospital, by way of the street, to the college building. All of the way I kept talking about her confidence in you and the success of the operation, but offered no explanation for leaving the hospital. I suppose she thought it was the usual procedure."

I was talking against time, waiting eagerly, but with uncertainty, for the sound of the operating table as it rolled over the floor on its way to the pit. Fortune, faith and good luck were with me. The operating table came rumbling in, and nothing else mattered. I was master of the situation, and began the operation.

At this juncture, Dr. Mary McEwen, my able and dependable first assistant, whispered in my ear, "They want to see you in the room just outside the pit."

I flouted the idea. "Say that I am conducting a clinic, and cannot be disturbed."

With a look from her that I respected, she begged, "Do go!"

I paused. "All right, but you'll have to go on with the clinical lecture until I return. And don't stop on any account."

I slid out of the pit, and asked the waiting college superintendent, "What can I do for you?"

He demanded, "Where are you going to take this patient after the operation?"

"Where she will get good care."

"As superintendent of the college, I cannot allow you to operate, and I have been instructed to tell you so."

"Well," I said, "you have certainly done as instructed. I think no one can put any blame on your shoulders."

I returned to the pit, and began the long operation, finishing at just three o'clock, the hour when the president of the hospital staff was to begin his surgical clinic. He was already there.

I took him aside and asked, "Where shall I take my patient? You have admitted her to the hospital, I have operated, and what next?"

He replied, "I was surprised to find the doors of the passageway locked. I think this matter has gone a little too far. But—you had better call an ambulance, and have the patient taken to the Woman's Hospital." Ten miles away on the South Side!

Inasmuch as there seemed to be nothing else to do, I called the ambulance, and went with the patient to the Woman's Hospital. I have often wondered whether she thought it strange to walk a block from the hospital to the operating room, undergo a long, difficult operation, and wake up in a hospital ten miles away, on another side of the city. She never made any remarks, and I never gave any explanation. She undoubtedly thought that it was all included in a free clinic operation.

I went to Dr. Quine, who interpreted the situation. "They have never been willing for you to hold a clinic in that pit. They do not want a woman surgeon on the faculty, and have watched for an opportunity to balk you. They have found it, and no matter how reasonable their talk, they will never give in."

I argued the matter. "There are only two more clinics before the college closes for the summer, and I can conduct them with ambulatory patients. As it will not be necessary to hold any clinics in the summer, I will have time to complete my program before the fall term, for I have no thought of giving up my position."

Day and night I thought of ways and means by which I might continue my clinic independently of the West Side Hospital, and it was not long before this plan crystallized. I could rent a vacant store across from the college and fit it up as a six-bed charity hospital with Miss Vincent as superintendent, Dr. McCollum resident physician, and a couple of nurses to assist in caring for the patients. I could get a hospital license because our nearest neighbor, the undertaker, would place at our disposal his morgue (necessary for hospital licensure), as well as his ambulance every Saturday morning to take the patients back and forth from our little hospital to the college amphitheater across the street.

When all details of the plan were perfected, I went with them to Dr. Quine. "I am not going to waste any time or energy fighting the hospital staff, unwarrantably prejudiced against me, but I have a plan of action."

When I told him of the new hospital setup, he was thrilled. Putting his arm about me and patting me on the head, with a look never to be forgotten, he baptized me, "Why little girl, I thought you were dead. You are just born."

The pangs of birth had certainly been suffered, and the delivery had been far from normal, in fact, most pathological. But we had three months in which to get the Gyneceum (the name we gave our little hospital) started.

The wards were fitted with black iron hospital beds and other furniture of mission type. The walls were painted dark green, with a white ceiling brought down low upon the sides to lessen the height of the store walls. The woodwork was painted black, and the effect was heightened by bedspreads and table covers of coarse Russian linen and a number of plaster bas-reliefs, one of which was a large Winged Victory put in a most conspicuous place. The store window was a problem, but we finally framed it in dark green denim curtains, with sash curtains of dark green silk. A mattress with a green denim cover was fitted into the deep window seat, where we arranged many huge pillows covered with the same material. The furnishings were not pretentious, but had a charm that I have never found in any other hospital.

The sine qua non for the success of our hospital came to us during the summer. I happened to attend a clinic given by Dr. Emil Ries, head surgeon of the Chicago Post Graduate School and a wonderful teacher, who in a few words explained a new kind of anesthetic called "twilight sleep". 1 learned the method of administration, and went again and again, until I understood and was confident that I could use this anesthetic in my new hospital. If I could, it would solve some of the vexing questions: would patients object to being carried in an ambulance, out of the hospital, across the street, up in an elevator, with students popping in and out at all times, to an anesthetizing room; would their relatives object when they heard the story with dramatic additions, from the patients; would the patients, if transported under ether anesthesia, not be running too great risks of post-operative pneumonia. All these difficulties might be settled by the use of this new anesthetic.

To introduce anything new, especially a new anesthetic, is not easy. My first difficulty was encountered when Miss Vincent, superintending nurse, a staunch friend and graduate of the Illinois Training School, told me with tears in her eyes, "I am sorry, but I dare not give the hypodermics to produce this anesthetic sleep."

Lest some accident occur, I took upon myself the responsibility of administering the twilight sleep. We worked feverishly all through the hot summer, but the opening of school in October found everything in readiness. The hour for my college clinic had been changed from one in the afternoon to eight in the morning, in order to avoid a clash with other clinics. Alice regarded the change as advantageous. She predicted, "People dislike getting up in the morning, even for deviltry."

To have the patients under twilight sleep for an eight o'clock clinic, I would rise a little past three, harness Kit, and drive twelve miles to the West Side. Then I would prepare and administer the initial hypodermic injection. After the first dose I was glad to take a nap, if only for three-quarters of an hour; then I prepared and gave the second dose. Next came breakfast, then the third dose, followed by a visit to the college amphitheater to prepare for the clinic.

In January the weather was very cold, and when I arrived one Saturday morning a little after four, with hands too cold to blanket the horse that would have to stand in front of the hospital until between ten and eleven o'clock, my conscientious and warmhearted nurse, Miss Vincent, gave in and promised, "From now on I will assume the responsibility, and give the hypodermics for the twilight sleep."

Dr. McCollum, my loyal friend, was acting as resident and anesthetist. She entered into the spirit of the fight, and though at first we worked with the new anesthetic in fear and awe, we soon found it a miracle-worker for our hospital. After the patient had been given the third hypodermic injection, she was so deeply asleep that, without resistance or cognizance, she was taken to the college amphitheater. Noise along the route, even in the college halls and elevator, fell on deaf ears. Still sleeping, she was prepared for operation, and examined in a most thorough manner by several students. After the operation she was taken back to our hospital, continuing to sleep until around noon. She awakened happy that her operation was over and that she felt so well. In the afternoon her relatives came and showered us with congratulations and praise for our care, and her excellent condition.

The day that Dr. Quine interviewed me about the position of Clinical Professor of Gynecology, he stressed the importance of the wealth of material needed to conduct an operative clinic at a specified hour every week, year in and year out. The full force of his dictum came to me many times that first summer.

As Mother had felt lost since Father's death, I planned to spend the Fourth of July with her on the farm. It was not without great trepidation for my clinic that I did so, although Dr. McEwen was on the ground to keep things in hand while I was away. I expected to return on Friday, the day before the clinic, for which I had arranged to operate on a patient who had been suffering from deep tears of the womb and perineum since the delivery of her four children, all instrumental births.

After my arrival at the farm a terrible storm washed away the bridge over the creek. This alarmed me lest I might not be able to get back to Chicago, and so I returned, luckily, two days before I had intended to do so.

I found Dr. McEwen in great distress because the patient who was to be operated on at the Saturday clinic had sent in word that she would have to postpone her operation.

When I saw the patient in the dispensary on Thursday, I at once realized that she was suffering from fear of the operation, even though she insisted that the only thing that disturbed her was her four children for whom she had no one to care while she was in the hospital. I was sure that if she gave way to this unconfessed fright, she might never have the operation and become, thereby, invalided for the rest of her life.

I was prepared and reconciled to assume the responsibility for everything and everybody when I operated in the college clinic, but I was not prepared to take on this added responsibility of the patient's family while she was in the hospital. However, rising to the occasion, I promised, "I will call for you tomorrow morning and we will find a place for the children."

We crowded the children into the buggy and visited institution after institution on the South Side, but none would take the little boy. There was one institution, fortunately, where they would take the two girls, and we left them there. Finally the mother decided to leave the boy at home with the oldest girl. I could not blame the mother for being worried, and to reassure her I offered to take her to the West Side Hospital Saturday morning. When I called, I found that she was not even ready and intended to put off the operation for a week lest the little boy catch cold. When I promised to see the little boy every day and, of more importance, impressed upon her the fact that the operation involved no risk to her life, she became composed and went with me to the hospital.

Leaving her there, I hurried back home, twelve miles, to spend an hour brushing up for the clinical lecture that must accompany the operation. But I was no sooner in the house than the telephone rang and the nurse shouted, "Your patient has left the hospital!"

I faltered, "If the patient should happen to return, call me at once."

Now what was I to lecture about? What was I to do? At the height of my despair the telephone rang again, and this time the nurse restored my optimism. "Your patient has returned!"

I directed, "Put the patient to bed, hide her clothing, and watch her until I arrive."

I got into the buggy, and drove as quickly as possible to the hospital, hitched the horse, and went to the patient, who was in great spirits. I explained, "A strange man will take you to the operating room, and a woman doctor will put you under an anesthetic. I will be close by, washing my hands. You will not see me, but I will be there."

I thought I had prepared her for any event, and was in the midst of the clinical lecture when Dr. McEwen, in a voice of suppressed excitement muttered, "They want you in the anesthetizing room at once."

"Oh!" I wrung my hands in agony. "Why did I ever try to operate on this woman!" I felt sure that she had died under the anesthetic, leaving those four young children, when, after all, the operation was not necessary for saving life. Many chances had been offered me to postpone the operation, or give it up altogether, and if I had accepted any one of them, I might have been saved this horrible disaster. I felt like a murderer or a kidnapper who had lured her victim to her death.

In a minute I was at the door of the anesthetizing room, and heard a loud voice giving vent to the most lurid, vulgar oaths that I had ever heard. Opening the door, I saw my patient in the middle of the floor, her leggings down around her ankles, and her short operating gown just above her waist, waving her arms above her head. The two men students and Dr. Orton, the anesthetist, had sought shelter in the corner of the room.

When I spoke the patient's name, she turned with a silly look, tried to pull down the short gown, and rushing to me, embraced me and gurgled in a sheepish voice, "Why, I've been wondering where you were." At a word from me, she hopped upon the table and was soon asleep. When she embraced me, her breath had revealed that after reaching the hospital she had gone out to get a nip. The nip had restored her shaken spirits, but had freed her from inhibition as well.

At one time when six patients had signed up for the Saturday clinic, and I was studying how to manage them most wisely and thriftily, they faded within forty-eight hours, one by one, into promises for another day. The last patient failed us just twelve hours before clinic time. Yet, four hours before the clinic an interesting rare emergency entered the hospital, and two hours later, another patient that we had expected the month before. In the eight years that we conducted the clinic, we never ran out of operative patients.

Every year—yes, every month—my appetite for teaching medicine, conducting free clinics and instructing nurses and interns was whetted, even though clinical and teaching appointments had to be made on time, and thus increased my difficulties in keeping up a large general practice. Still I was growing stronger in diagnosis and rapidly building up my surgical practice.

Just at this time, during the first ten years of the twentieth century, I began interrupting my practice every three months to visit the Mayo Clinic.

Nothing ever helped me in a professional way so much as a visit to that great clinic where I could see the best surgical technique in the world, and learn the principles of practical surgery from masters.

In Rochester I spent mornings watching operations and listening to lectures that I have never forgotten; afternoons, discussing with the visiting physicians the operated cases.

Never have I met anyone from whom I was able to learn more, and having found the greatest surgical teacher in the world, I planned to go again soon to spend a week. My second experience was even happier than my first and after that I visited the Mayo Clinic every three months, staying a week each time. I continued this habit year after year until my appointment on the staff of the Cook County Hospital in 1913 made it impossible.

The very air of Rochester was rural and restful. No visiting physician was ever seen rushing from the Mayo Clinic to attend some other, to be on time for a dinner engagement, or to see a show. The place was brimful and running over with surgery, and there was time enough for it to soak in

Dr. William Mayo often punctuated his lectures by reciting incidents that were typically "Mayoesque." In the middle of an operation I saw him stop, and request that the patient's history be reread. After listening attentively, he gave the reason for the delay. "Patients always have some symptoms from which they wish relief. Their interest is not how many organs are removed, but whether the operation will relieve their symptoms."

Warning against the habit of criticizing subordinates, he told of a surgeon in New York City, who always called down first one nurse or intern and then another for the slightest slip in technique. One morning, as this New York surgeon made the initial incision for a herniotomy, he cut more deeply than he had intended and accidentally opened into the bowel itself. Dr. Mayo, who was a spectator, chuckled at the thought that this time he could find no one to blame except himself. But no—quick as a wink he turned to the nurse with these accusing words: "Now, see what you have made me do—you give me a butter knife for three months, and then a razor, without warning!"

Dr. Will emphasized the danger in making a hasty diagnosis of neurasthenia in obscure cases. He related the case of a well-to-do patient who came to the clinic. "I do not wish to imply that the insides of well-to-do patients are different from others, but that she had had a great amount of medical attention. She went through our clinic, where no disease was discovered, and was discharged after the prescribing of a tonic.

"On the way to her home in the South she stopped in Cincinnati, and consulted the doctor of one of her friends. He sent her to the hospital, and removed a gallstone as big as a walnut. The patient sent us the stone with a letter that no lady would write." Dr. Mayo shook his head and continued, "Since then we have never dismissed a patient with a diagnosis of neurasthenia in order to cover our inability to find out and cure her disease."

The trials and tribulations of the great are often the support and stimulus of the weak. While struggling with my clinic in the University of Illinois College of Medicine, I heard a story of the Mayo brothers that almost made me feel akin to those great surgeons and teachers.

This story I learned from a barber, when spending a week at the Mayo Clinic. While shampooing my hair, so long and heavy that I needed entertainment during the drying, he told a tale of the very early days when the Mayo Clinic was in an embryonic state. Dr. Will was operating and Dr. Charlie was assisting. They had just finished one operation and begun another, when word came from the ward that the first patient was dead. They completed the second operation, but before they had started their third, the second patient expired. The fourth patient was brought to the operating room, but the third passed out as he was being taken from the operating room, and the fourth died on the table.

Dr. Will sat down, and looked at Dr. Charlie. "Charlie," he said, "we can keep this up for a while, but not for long. We might as well quit now, and go back to the farm and get to work."

"But," the barber chuckled, his eyes shining as he winked at me, "they never did."

This may be a fictitious story that the Mayo brothers never heard, or it may be true, but if it is, only such courageous geniuses as they could have withstood this crucial ordeal.

13

THE BEGINNINGS OF SEX EDUCATION

BECAUSE I was devoting so much of my time to teaching and conducting free clinics, I did not feel that I could spare a minute for social activities. When one of my grateful patients took no end of trouble to make me a member of the Chicago Woman's Club, I was dismayed rather than pleased. My patient paid my initiation fee (one hundred dollars) and the dues for that year. She intended to give me a happy surprise, for at that time it was difficult to become a member, but the surprise would have been on her if she could have known that I looked upon this membership as a tempting apple, the eating of which might drive me from my paradise, the practice of medicine.

When I enrolled in the Home Department of the Club, every one was amazed, but it mattered little what group I was identified with, for I never attended any meetings.

It was a real surprise when I found that I could work for the club in the capacity of a woman physician. Social hygiene and sex education for children came to life at the beginning of the twentieth century, but for many years had to be handled with art and subterfuge. The Committee on Social Purity, inaugurated in 1907, was made up of the most womanly women in the Club, and it was this committee that asked the women physicians, members of the Club, to give a course of lectures on sex.

Drs. Anna Blount, Harriet Barringer Alexander, Caroline Hedger, Alice Barlow Brown, Josephine Young, Rose Erlanger, Rachelle Yarrows and I composed the group. Each doctor had the privilege of selecting the subject of her own lecture. I had never lectured to any lay group except at the Armour Institute where I had given instruction in First Aid. I felt too inexperienced to speak on any sex problem, but I was so sure of myself in the field of anatomy that I suggested, "I might tell them something about the anatomy and physiology of the sexual organs, male and female."

"Fine," they chorused, "and that subject is so fundamental that you must give the first lecture."

At once I saw what a predicament I had wished on myself. If my audience did not like the talk, they would never return to listen to the really fine lectures of my colleagues.

I was worried and spent many days writing out speeches only to tear them up. There were many angles to the problem: my audience must not be made to feel sex conscious; they must be made to admire the anatomical sexual structures; they must be made to understand my sex vocabulary; and most important, they must never be allowed to be shocked or disgusted. All these points were flapping before my mind, like a Monday's wash on a sagging clothesline, when I thought of a simple device, that would help me out of my difficulties, as a strong clothes pole prevents the snowy garments from falling to the ground.

I would illustrate my talk by first drawing on the blackboard, the sexless sexual organs of a three-months-old fetus, a baby six months before birth, and from this indifferent fundament develop, by sketches, the female organs to the right, and the male organs to the left. My audience would be introduced to embryology, and charmed by its mystery, led unconsciously into the beauties and miracles of sex.

This first lecture would be the test in immunizing my audience to shock and embarrassment to the end that they would eagerly return for the lectures to follow: Sex Education for Children; Adolescent Problems; Marriage Advice; The Menopause; Dangers of Syphilis; Gonorrhoea, a Contageous Disease; and Sex Psychology.

We lectured in the Public Library, the small-park club houses, the Memorial Hospital, and the parlors of the Chicago Woman's Club, to audiences of mothers and children, club women and working girls. Eight lectures, one by each member of the doctors' group, were given many times to constantly increasing and enthusiastic listeners.

The Club appreciated our work and appointed charming, gracious hostesses to introduce the speakers. Mrs. Charles Henrotin, president of the Club in 1903, always introduced me. There was a French lilt to her voice and a French tang to her clothes that shed a radiance upon my direct Dutch approach and, I am sure, improved my talk, or at least the audience's reception of it.

One day, after I had finished and we were about to leave, she said, "As many times as I have heard you speak on this same subject, I am never bored and, at the close, I stand spellbound, looking at your audience. They are wrapped in admiration over the drawing on the board—as if they were of rare and beautiful flowers instead of testicles, ovaries, penises, scrotums, and wombs."

In 1912, after five years of social hygiene lecturing that kindled the fires of a revolution in sex education, the Chicago Woman's Club came to the conclusion that instruction in sex hygiene should be given over to the teaching profession. Soon after this decision Ella Flagg Young, Superintendent of Chicago Public Schools from 1909 to 1915, assigned a large group of Chicago men and women physicians to give lectures at certain schools on sex hygiene.

I was asked to assist in choosing the individuals for this group of medical men and women whom she addressed before they began their talks. Mrs. Young gave clear-cut instructions: "Use such language that the children will understand you, but say nothing that will bring a blush to the cheek of the most reticent, innocent girl. We have invited all of the parents and many will be there. What you say must not shock them, or suggest anything coarse or vulgar—"

She had a deep-toned voice that she could lower in a most impressive manner. Her words came slowly: ". . . But you must tell them everything."

The Senn High School was assigned to me. With many misgivings I faced my audience of two hundred senior girls. Scores of parents were seated at the back of the room.

Hoping to become immediately intimate with my audience, I began in story-telling fashion, "Once upon a time when each of you in this room was no bigger than my thumb—" At this point, as I extended my uplifted thumb towards my listeners, I noticed the face of a girl in the front row take on a sickly pallor. I was determined that no child should faint, and in desperation, regardless of the continuity of my talk, I rapidly created a diversion. "Why my thumb is dirty! I compared it to you!" I made a low bow. "Forgive me, children; I know none of you ever had dirty hands!" At this point the children laughed, and the pink came stealing back into the cheeks of the girl in the front row. I proceeded cautiously, watching the faces of the children and interspersing my speech as the occasion demanded with remarks intended to be amazing, amusing, or just irrelevant, until the blackboard was covered with drawings of testicles, ovaries, sperm cells, ova, oviducts, external genitals—all made during the talk to illustrate the development and function of the sexual organs, male and female.

No girl fainted, but before I finished I could have swooned from exhaustion. The teacher graciously complimented me. "It was fine. I really enjoyed it, though at first I was afraid one little girl was going to faint. In fact, we expected that, and had made everything ready for such an emergency."

Difficult as they were, the sex hygiene lectures given in the Chicago public schools were not to be compared with the ones I gave later at Oxford College in Ohio.

The dean of the school, whom I had known when she was

studying for her Ph.D. degree at the University of Michigan, called at the office and announced, "I understand you can talk to young women about sex hygiene without upsetting them."

I replied, "I should hope so."

Forthwith we laid plans and settled the time and remuneration for a trip to Oxford, Ohio. Inadvertently, Dean Sherzer remarked, "A few years ago a woman doctor gave them a talk, and we haven't dared to mention the subject since."

"Oh! My dear Dean! In that case we must make a complete change in our line of conduct. If you have had a speaker so tactless that she has raped her audience, the only course for me is to seduce them."

Then I formulated this program: "I will arrive in the morning just in time for your morning exercises and will give a talk on Women in Medicine. At lunch you can announce that you have persuaded me to remain over till a late train, and in the afternoon I will tell them what the Chicago Woman's Club is doing for Chicago's betterment."

After a flattering introduction, I stood before my audience of bright young girls and wondered what my predecessor could have said to have disturbed them so seriously. In my vocational talk I described a dinner that the Chicago women doctors gave each month. I told anecdotes about women specialists in eye and ear, surgery, pediatrics and other branches of medicine, all recognized as successful professionally and financially.

In conclusion I struck the keynote. "Perhaps you picture the woman doctor going from house to house, in all kinds of weather, day and night, to visit sick and dying patients. That describes a general practitioner, the role I played for fifteen years—years so precious to me that I would forego any reward I have received as a specialist for one of them."

Then I gave a melodramatic description of a woman doctor's "My Day". Rushing from an emergency delivery of a premature baby to operate on a ruptured appendix, keeping crowded office hours that are held up by a sudden death, driving miles to make house calls, and taking no time for her meals, the doctor is left at midnight sitting by the crib of a baby suffering with pneumonia. The crisis of the disease comes at daybreak.

I paused, for some of the girls were sobbing, and all were deeply moved. "Thank you! I see that every one of you feels with me. The best reward of the practice of medicine is not fame or fortune, but the opportunity to render human service."

Later I asked the dean, "Why were your girls disturbed by the woman doctor who spoke to them several years ago?" I received no explanation. I insisted on an answer and declared that I would not leave town until this mystery was cleared.

Hesitatingly, with bowed head and flaming cheeks, the dean related how my predecessor had made use of two dolls to demonstrate the technique of sexual relations. I was at first shocked—then smiled, when I pictured the earnest and worried doctor who, in her zeal "to tell everything," as Superintendent Ella Flagg Young had admonished, had forgotten that animal instinct could be depended upon long before speech or the alphabet came into being. The preservation of the human race is too serious to be left to haphazard, and needs no dramatization. On later consideration I have grieved that she missed the golden opportunity to thrill those adolescents with the real miracle of life.

An unlighted open fireplace, little more than a pile of wood and kindling, is a place in which children may play safely until a burning match is applied to it. Then the inert mass is transformed into a flaming source of heat and light; a hazard to those who ignorantly would handle it. I like to compare the grate, piled high with unburned logs, to sex education from which no damage can come until the igniting match of sex awakening kindles a fire—a force that demands understanding to curb and direct its heat.

The import of sex awakening in the education of children was forcefully brought out by the wife of the Superintendent of the Illinois State Normal School at a luncheon meeting of the Parents and Teachers State Association in Springfield, Illinois. She corroborated my speech in which I stressed the importance of non-interference with children in their self-directed efforts to acquire sex information.

Her talk ran in this wise: "I have three boys, the oldest, up to the age of twelve, had been delicate, and had had a tutor at home. Since our son was to enter public school in the fall, and we were planning to spend the summer in our house on the bank of one of Wisconsin's beautiful lakes, I asked my husband if he did not think it would be wise for him to take our son for a walk in the woods and give him a little talk about life; sex information might come better from his father than from his schoolmates. My husband, feeling that it was the duty of the father to instruct his son, acquiesced completely.

"Quite unexpectedly, not more than an hour after our arrival at the summer home, our oldest son rushed into the house, upstairs to his room, and threw himself upon the bed, weeping convulsively. Hurriedly following him, I inquired as to the cause of his grief. In a shrill voice he ordered me out of his room. 'You do it too—you and Father—I hate you both.'

"It seems that the daughter of our nearest neighbor, a minister, had in that first brief hour told him all she knew about sex. The talk that my husband was to give our son began at once, and continued day after day. Sex always has remained a distasteful subject to my son, and even after he had finished college, he confessed to reliving at times that terrible day when sex knowledge was first brought to him.

"Not wishing to duplicate this tragic mistake, I at once resolved to instruct my son of eight. I studied and hunted for honeyed words with which I might make the story of life a simple tale fit for the ears of an innocent little boy. When I had learned my speech, my mouth dry from nervousness, I asked my small son to sit on the stool at my feet, and listen to what Mother had to tell him. He looked up at me with such an angelic expression that I had to force myself to talk. When I reached the end, he bowed his head, and spoke slowly. 'Mother, won't you be very angry if I tell you something?' I was already repaid by this burst of confidence.

"No, my son, I won't be angry. I want you to tell me everything that is in your mind."

" 'Well,' he confessed, 'I have known all that for a long time.' I gasped—again I was too late.

"We had still another son, a boy of four. We never told him in so many words anything about sex, but on the other hand, nothing was ever kept from him. He has been one with us and of us. When he asks questions, we answer him directly and truthfully, and if we talk over his head, his curiosity is not even excited, for he knows we have no secrets from him. He is the only one of my sons normally educated in regard to sex matters."

Sex education for children, begun by visual demonstrations for small children, should not be considered complete until the child reaches the age of sexual awakening. There is little doubt that no information is more desired then that pertaining to sex; yet, in spite of its universal appeal, sex education, as such, is not recognized even in medical schools.

The eagerness for books that refer unblushingly to sex conditions and situations is a pitiful demonstration of the hunger on the part of the public for anything connected with genesis. Ignorance on no other subject could be more productive of bad results—illegitimacy, child murder, veneral diseases, abortion, divorce, suicide, and homicide.

In a practice that is ninety per cent gynecology and obstetrics, it often becomes imperative to give advice in regard to the sexual life of the individual. In this role I became familiar with the usual, customary and habitual sex habits not only of the married but of the unmarried as well. Giving marital advice and hunting for the causes of symptoms of disease, I unearthed most distressing conditions.

I was instructing a patient that marital relations must not be resumed for two months after her operation when she scoffed, "Well then, I will have to stay at the hospital for two months."

"I, myself, will speak to your husband."

"Hah! That would make no difference; he comes home every noon, and I have to submit to him." She continued, "Why he's even sorry that I have never slept with other men and so cannot appreciate what a wonderful screw he is."

I had been in private practice less than five years when there came to the clinic a young woman with a complete laceration of the perineum, resulting in complete inability to control the bowel movements. I had been so successful with this, my solo operation at the New England Hospital for Women and Children, that I was eager and felt able to perform an operation to cure her. The patient was indigent, but I succeeded in securing a charity bed, and offered to operate gratis.

She shook her head, and with sad wistfulness asserted, "My husband would never consent."

"I will ask him, and explain it all," I reassured her, and that evening I called at the house, and delivered a speech that I guaranteed to move the stoniest heart of the most obdurate male.

This husband looked at me with an expression that brought panic to my heart, and blushes to my cheeks. He blurted, "Naw, naw, 'twould be no good. I'd bust her first time I ust her."

Nauseated, and with those terrible words grating on my ear, I groped my way to the back porch, and leaning over the railing, I parted with my good supper. I never saw my poor prostituted patient or her callous husband again, but their memory clings to me like the odor of a repulsive disease.

There were many great businessmen, lawyers, ministers and doctors whose wives had poured into my ears extravagant tales of sex deviation from normal standards.

During the last two decades stories of sexual atrocities in married life have not crept into our office histories. In their place are unbelievable examples of sexual control and consideration.

The best illustration of the changing times was a visit of a fifty-year-old mother with her daughter, who had been married two years. The mother wanted to see me first and privately. Glancing around to make sure that we were alone, she informed me in a very confidential voice, "Now, my daughter is not well, and these young people—you know—at it all the time. She can't stand it. Please, you tell her—you know—they must go a little more moderate. You can tell her."

The daughter was then admitted, and when I made a pelvic examination, I put the question, "You are still a virgin; is there any reason for it?"

The mother's eyes grew large; her mouth opened wide; then followed unbelievable accusations. "What are you up to? Don't you know anything? Do you want to send your husband to houses of prostitution? Have you lost your mind?"

I interrupted, and begged her to allow me to talk with her daughter. She left us, muttering, "Well, did you ever? What are we coming to?"

With the mother out of hearing the daughter laid the facts before me. "My husband and I had a long engagement. His salary was smaller than mine, but when he got a good raise, he wanted to get married, and thought I should not work as my health was failing. After we were married, he said, 'I guess married life takes something out of you; how would it be if we went right along just as we did before we were married, until you are well and strong?' It was all right with me, and that's all there is to it. Is there anything wrong about it?"

"No—but I advise you to rely upon your husband. He is modern, and your mother—well, perhaps too Victorian for a twentieth-century adviser."

At another time a patient consulted me for persistent hemorrhages caused by a large fibroid tumor. I advised her, "You are going to have that large growth removed. When do you want the operation?"

She replied emphatically, "Never!"

I continued, "You do not have to have me perform the operation—but it must be done by someone at once—the only question for you to answer is what day, and that day must be within a week."

She remained obdurate, finally confiding the real reason for not wanting the operation. "You see, my husband and I have a most satisfactory and delightful sexual life. When we were first married, he said to me, 'Now I know very little about these things, but I do know that all males are ready at any time, whereas females have desires only at certain periods. Since I cannot tell when this may be acceptable to you, I will never suggest such a thing. Knowing that I am always ready, the approach will be entirely in your hands.' I have had my family, and in all my nearly thirty years of married life he has never made a demand, and I would rather die than have our marital relations disturbed."

I easily convinced her that the tumor, and not an operation, would endanger her sex life, and she consented to the operation.

Mutual, voluntary, marital continence, not forced by impotence or frigidity, has come to my knowledge many times, so many that I look upon the present generation with unbounded admiration.

In June 1934, at the fiftieth reunion of my literary class in the University of Michigan, I voiced my feelings. We had had our banquet, the speeches that followed, and were sitting around the table engaging in small-group conversation when one of the twenty-five men present called out, "I can't understand why Bertha never married. When we graduated, I would have wagered that she would be the first girl."

"I, too," came from a dozen of the listeners. Then one inquired, "Why didn't you?"

All eyes were upon me, but my blushing days were over. I hesitated, "Would you really like to know? Wouldn't you be offended if I told you?"

"No! No! Tell us." It was unanimous.

"Well," I retorted, "if the boys when I was of a marriageable age had been like the boys of today, I would have set up a male harem."

Everyone gasped, and one spoke slowly, "You mean we were not good enough?"

I nodded assent.

MOTHER WON A RACE

THERE WERE no lavatories on the North African train, and as it took two days to go from Algiers to Biskra, it was necessary occasionally to search for one. I have seen a great many races—horse races, dog races, chariot races in the circus, foot races among college men, races at county fairs where they have the three-legged races and the potato races, but I never saw anything so laughable as the race between my Mother and an Arab to see who could get first to the outdoor toilet above five hundred feet from the train at one of the stops.

Mother's hair was snowy white, and she wore black, with a long widow's veil. The Arab had his black head bound with a white turban, and his long white burnoose that came to his heels, was so wide that it surrounded him like a cloud as he raced along. Mother's eighty-year-old legs had half a century of training on the farm, and she was gaining steadily on the Arab. Then too, she knew how to take the uneven ground. We laughed till we were helpless when she finally took the prize, a seat in the backhouse!

14

EUROPE AND NORTH AFRICA

FROM THE BEGINNING, my medical career, like a many-lobed placenta, was the medium through which everything that sustained me must filter. I took no vacations, never read the newspapers, limited my reading to medicine, and seldom allowed my thoughts to wander far from my professional duties. Alice would frequently say, "You aren't listening to me!" At times I would be too deep in thought to get off at my station on the elevated road, occasionally passing it two or three times.

When after a couple of months of especially confining work, a let-up came, I indulged myself by lunching at the Chicago Woman's Club, at that time seven blocks from my office. .I left the club at one o'clock to return to the office, but oblivious of the passage of time, window-shopped all the way back. Nearing Field's, I looked at the clock—it was four—I had spent three hours going seven blocks! It was unbelievable! As I entered the office, the attendant anxiously inquired, "What happened?"

I shook my head and whispered, "Terrible!"

"I knew it," she said. 'I have just had to sit down on the patients for the past hour."

I continued shaking my head, and began getting rid of a roomful of restless people. I murmured frequently, "So sorry!" and the episode ended. A year passed before I dared to tell my office lady of what I had been guilty. When I had finished, she grated her teeth. "Even now I have half a mind to beat you!" she threatened.

It was also during these busy years that my desire for culture prompted me to buy a season ticket for the opera. The dates conflicted so much with sick duties that I gave most of the tickets to friends. However, I made the grade one night, and was very happy when the curtain rose, and the musical drama began. But—the next thing I knew, Alice was poking me in the ribs, saying, "You'd better wake up if you want to see the killing."

I had slept through the entire opera, including the intermissions. After that I recommended grand opera for insomnia—pleasant, effectual, and no leftovers.

Although I love to window-shop, I can manage to walk many blocks in record-breaking time, past the most seductive windows. One notable example was when Isadora Duncan made her appearance at Orchestra Hall in Chicago. Alice urged me to buy tickets in advance to see the much applauded dancer, but as the performance conflicted with my office hours, I would not consider it. Nevertheless, when the day came, I weakened. Having no ticket, and too late to buy a reserved seat, I determined to go early, and fight with the mob for a seat in the gallery. I saw a few patients before leaving my office, and rushing five blocks to the hall, stood nearly half an hour before the doors opened. Then I hopped, skipped and jumped up five flights of stairs, down the long gallery steps, and quickly secured a seat in the center wedge, three rows from the front. I left my bag and coat on a seat, and galloping back up the gallery steps, and down the many flights of stairs, I retraced the five blocks to the office, where I saw waiting patients as fast as they would allow me. At two-thirty again I hied myself to Orchestra Hall. This time I ran the five blocks, climbed the five flights, two steps at a time, and groping my way, found my belongings safe, and every seat occupied except this one that I had recklessly reserved by leaving my possessions upon it.

I had no program, but it mattered little, for every number

was by Duncan herself, and the encores were many. Time never passed more quickly—all eyes riveted on her every movement. Her feet and arms were bare, and she wore only a simple Grecian tunic which she did not change during the entire performance. Under her spell it seemed that classic figures, one by one, stepped forth from painted decorations on urns and vases, or from the sculptured surface of a frieze, and lambent with ecstasy of life, were moving about the stage. Her audience held her like a passionate lover who refuses to say good-by. When at last she would not give another encore, or even take a bow, the spellbound crowd remained in their seats. The orchestra climbed over the footlights, and the stage was empty. Still the applause continued. After it died away, the people sat like hypnotic subjects, unable to move. A quarter of an hour had elapsed since Duncan had withdrawn before any movement to leave began, but finally that concourse came back to earth, and slowly left the hall. A man whom I did not know, turned to me, and said almost incredulously, "Really, I thought I had seen dancing, but I never had."

Sarah and I have never cared to dance; nevertheless, no other entertainment gives me the emotional appeal that a terpsichorean one affords. During one of Pavlova's visits to Chicago, I sated myself with seeing her in eight consecutive performances in one week. Since then, whenever I hear Paderewski's minuet, I close my eyes and see Pavlova, that miracle of motion, in an Empire gown, its train caught to her wrist, a tall poke bonnet framing her pallid face.

To leave one's medical practice with a competent and loyal colleague aceptable to patients, and make preparations for everybody's comfort and pleasure during even a short holiday, often entails an expenditure of energy sufficient to nullify all of its benefits. Such reasons had influenced me against taking any vacations since I began practice eighteen years before.

There were, however, many reasons for taking a long vacation at this time. My niece's fight with diabetes insipidus for the past ten years had kept her from being so sophisticated as most girls of her age. Accordingly, Alice and I thought it would be well for her to postpone entering college and substitute a year of travel for a deficiency in social training. Mother, in her eightieth year, was so well and strong that I was sure she would enjoy seeing the Old World. Moreover, Alice needed a change. Consequently, plans were laid to sail in July, 1909, on the steamship Ionia from Montreal to Glasgow, Scotland.

All the vacation travels I have ever taken have had a very definite purpose, a sort of focal point in the guise of a medical meeting. I am sure I should have felt like a Sister of the Road, Box Car Bertha, if I had not had a medical meeting as the ostensible reason for taking a trip. By this time Alice had been to so many medical meetings with me that she took a firm stand on that subject. "When you want to take a vacation, I am ready to go with you, but I am never going to any more medical meetings." Consequently, while laying plans I talked more of the trip itself, putting the meetings in as by-products, in order not to have to leave Alice at home.

This time I was going to read a paper on "The Effect of Scopolamine Morphine Anesthesia on the Fetus in Utero," at the Sixteenth International Medical Congress, in Budapest, Hungary, the second week of September, 1909.

In order to read a paper at this meeting, I had had to make application and send in the subject one year before the Congress. On May 15, of that same year, I received notification of its acceptance. I then sent a check for my entertainment while in Budapest.

Although I have embarked on twenty-two ships since we sailed up the St. Lawrence River and out into the Atlantic Ocean on the one-class Scottish steamship Ionia, none of them has made such a lasting impression on me as that first boat. While still on the river, we read our telegrams and letters, and enjoyed the view through the beautiful binoculars that were given me by my students in the same amphitheater where, eight years before, the dean had been called to quell the riot against me.

Since the North Atlantic route is short, it was not long before we sailed up the Firth of Forth. In Edinburgh I met Dr. Elsie Inglis, who took me to the Edinburgh Infirmary to see Dr. Alexis Thompson, distinguished Scotch surgeon, operate. We were already seated in the amphitheater when Dr. Thompson entered the operating arena. Dr. Inglis leaned forward and whispered to me, "Does Dr. Mayo wear his collar and necktie when operating?"

"Never," I replied.

A few minutes later she contined, "Does Dr. Mayo always wear rubber gloves?"

"Yes, always," I said.

And again, "Does Dr. Mayo wear his street trousers, or does he wear white ones?"

"White ones," and I began to be curious at the questions.

Later she explained her queries. "Dr. Alexis Thompson has recently visited America and the Mayo clinic, but before he went, he never removed his collar or necktie, in preparation for an operation. He wore street trousers and often, no rubber gloves. Since his return, he always takes off collar, tie and street clothing, changes to white trousers, and always wears rubber gloves."

Dr. Inglis arranged for me to operate in her own hospital on High Street, and also in the Woman's Hospital. To the operations in the Woman's Hospital she invited women physicians from Glasgow, Aberdeen, Rumbling Bridge and Perth, as well as physicians in Edinburgh. Following the operating we had tea, at which Dr. Johnston, an old friend and patient, presided.

Dr. Inglis invited the out-of-town guests and me to her home for dinner that night. While I was dressing for the party, Dr. Johnston called and I asked her, "Is there anything I ought or ought not to do tonight?"

She was amused. "Everything will be all right, but I wonder what you are going to wear?"

"My new tailored suit; it has a silk top, wool jumper skirt, and a short coat."

"That will be all right for you," she mused, "but don't be surprised if you see the rest of the guests with low neck and short or no sleeves."

To do in Scotland as the Scotch do, I dug out of the trunk a dress of golden brown grenadine over yellow silk, with low neck and short puffed sleeves. I had brought it as a formal for the medical meeting in Budapest, in September. "Would this do?"

"Just the right thing," she assured me.

During the dinner a call came for Dr. Inglis, who ordered a carriage, and in her evening dress covered by an opera cloak, made the visit and returned, having missed only one course. I wondered what my patients would think if I should attend them in such attire.

We left Scotland to cross Germany, Bohemia and Austria, making only very short stops because we expected to visit them on our return. From Vienna we went to Budapest by boat.

On arriving at Budapest, we hunted up convention headquarters, and found that we had been assigned rooms in a large school building in which beds and washstands had been installed. The blackboards and friezes of rolled-up maps, the wide empty corridors, the far-distant toilets, and bare windows all testified to the great difficulty Budapest had experienced in entertaining an international medical congress. Nevertheless these meager housing comforts only accentuated the zeal of the Hungarians as hosts, and in all Europe we never found a city so beautiful as Budapest, with its countless public statues set off by backgrounds of green trees. Compared with any other medical convention I have ever attended, it is still ultra.

At the palace a reception was given for the convention delegates by Emperor Franz Joseph. He did not appear in person, but was represented by the Crown Prince Ferdinand d'Este. We were surprised when Dr. Rosina Wistein, my Czechoslovakian friend who had been my pupil and assistant in my gynecological clinic in Chicago, would not go and gave her ticket to one of our party. At that time the hatred between Hungary and Bohemia was so great that Dr. Wistein would not accept a courtesy from the Austrian Emperor.

Dr. May Michael, a promising pediatrician from Chicago, her sister, and Alice and I, arrayed in our reception gowns, took a carriage and started for the palace. All went well until we reached the hill on which the palace had been built. At its foot our driver stopped and refused to go any farther. We thought it was because he did not understand, and in all the languages in which we could speak even a few words, we directed, "To the King's Palace."

He was immovable, and as a last resort Dr. Michael asked him to take us back to the hotel. "The head porter there can make him understand," she said.

With evident relief he returned us to the hotel, where the head porter quickly bade us get out of the carriage, and dismissing the driver, called another, assuring us that now there would be no difficulty. Before leaving, we insisted on knowing what had caused the trouble.

"Why," he laughed, "you were in a one-horse carriage, and only a two-horse carriage is allowed to go to the palace."

We finally got there and walked up the long steep flight of stairs leading to the entrance of the palace. We passed between cordons of gorgeously uniformed guards, and were conducted to a large empty room. We stared—the floor was covered with piles of folded-up coats and wraps! We folded up our coats and parked them in a row with the others.

Then doors were opened through which we entered into a room about forty feet square, without seats or furniture, where we stood or were pushed about among unintroduced strangers. From this room we advanced, room by room, until we reached the fifth, where, with aching feet and disillusionment about the joy of meeting royalty, we found ourselves in the presence of His Highness, the Crown Prince. After grasping his hand, we began the retreat, room by room, as we had advanced.

Everything was very dignified and orderly until waiters appeared with trays of food held high above their heads. At sight of the refreshments there was a grand barnyard-like scramble for the food. The guests leaped into the air and, before the food could be served, literally grabbed the drinks, sandwiches, and cakes from the trays, necessitating the waiters to return to the kitchens for more. When tray after tray was emptied before the waiters had advanced two feet, one of the Hungarian physicians snatched some food for us from a passing waiter's highborne tray.

Some of these experiences may have been of real value in assisting me through the ordeal of reading my paper. To go to the platform and read a paper sounds simple enough—but not in Budapest. The first day of the Congress I was given a program printed in English, according to which it would be impossible for my paper to be reached the first day. Consequently, I took a back seat and noted the conduct of the meeting. The next day I chose a seat nearer the front, and though my paper was not called, I was positive that it would be, early in the morning of the third day. Thereupon, with habits of promptness that I have never succeeded in modifying, I arrived at the lecture room just as the doors were thrown open. I had come without my breakfast and selected a seat in the first row, directly in front of the speaker's desk.

It was not long before one of the Hungarian secretaries came in. We chatted until the lecture room filled up, and four other secretaries arrived. When the clerk came, he began to write the morning's program on the blackboard, and I was surprised to find that he had omitted my name. At first I took it for granted that the order had been changed to accommodate some member of the Congress, but since no name had been put in place of mine, I consulted my newly made acquaintance.

"Are you going to read a paper?" he questioned, and I answered by pointing to my name and the subject of my paper on the printed program.

Going to the clerk, he talked with him until they were shouting excitedly and gesticulating wildly. When the Hungarian secretary returned, he gave directions, "Your paper comes right here in the program" (pointing to the name preceding mine). "Now when this gentleman has almost finished, go to the platform, and as he moves away, step right up, announce your subject and read your paper. Don't wait to be called."

The clerk, on his part, in a very small insignificant hand, wrote my name on the blackboard.

Up to this moment my legs and arms had been trembling in a most uncomfortable manner, but now my entire attitude changed. I saw that it was going to take more than a ladylike, modest, scientific bearing to read my paper. I began to feel like a bronco buster or a gentleman burglar, and no longer scared. When the doctor with the paper immediately preceding mine began to read, I sat bolt upright on the chair, my right foot stretched out in front of me, and with every page that the speaker turned down, I slipped farther towards the edge of my seat. I took on baseball tactics. With my hand still clutching my chair, I was creeping nearer the platform. When the speaker came to the last page, I had left my hold on the chair, and was crouching at the base of the speakers' stand. When the speaker was moving to leave, I was standing beside him. I announced my subject, and with the sureness of a victor I read my paper slowly and in a loud voice.

I left the platform in a din of applause, of which I had deprived my predecessor, and was surrounded by congratulatory friends. Foremost among them was Herr Professor Gauss, who, when he learned that I had never given scopolamine in obstetrical work, begged me to do so, saying, "You, more than any other person I know, have fitted yourself to give it."

It was great satisfaction to see that my paper was published in Munich before it was published in the United States.

After our Budapest experience we retraced our steps to Vienna where I had expected to spend most of my time in medical work. I began by attending a clinic in the Woman's Hospital, and was surprised when the patient, perfectly naked and conscious, was brought into the operating room on a bare metal cart. All the assistants and the surgeon himself wore high rubber boots, and the floor was swimming with water, for whenever any solution had to be renewed, the old one was spilled upon the floor! This was a new and startling technique to me. When the patient had been anesthetized and covered with a sterile sheet, the surgeon began an abdominal operation for the removal of a small tumor. He first opened the abdomen and made an apparently deliberate, but I know it was accidental, cut over an inch in length in the urinary bladder. He stopped, saw his mistake, and proceeded to sew up the bladder wound.

At dinner that night one of the half-dozen doctors at the table asked, "What have you done during the day?"

I bantered, "Completed a course in gynecological surgery," and related the case, but evidently gave offense by my sweeping criticism, for no one spoke.

The third day I attended the clinic of another celebrated Viennese surgeon. He was scheduled to begin early in the morning, but did not arrive until ten-thirty. Three patients, however, had been brought into the operating room: a woman about twenty years of age, an old man of sixty and a younger man of forty. They were all naked, all conscious, and lying on bare metal tables. When at long last the chief arrived, he selected the young woman first for operation, made an incision in her side seven inches in length, and removed a rather harmless looking appendix. The next patient was the old man. While he had been lying there waiting, looking full of vigor, I had wondered what disease he could be unfortunate enough to have. As soon as he was under the anesthetic, the sterile sheet was drawn over his legs and I said, sotto voce, "Not below the knees." As the sheet was hoisted higher up, "Above the waist." As the sheet continued to be drawn higher, "Oh, a head operation." The sheet halted just above the eyes, and the operation proved to be the removal of a small wart on the lower part of the forehead.

I made no remarks that night when I met my colleagues at dinner, but I listened with great interest as they told of the wonderful things they were learning, and of the great superiority of the post-graduate teaching in Vienna to that in the United States. Something was the matter with me, without a doubt. I was sure that I would get more out of hiking in the suburbs than by crowding into clinics.

In late autumn we went to Italy and from there to France where we spent Christmas. After the holidays we sailed for North Africa.

While in Algiers we saw our first bullfight. Arriving early, we watched the crowds assemble until every seat was full. After the impressive entrance of the matador and his followers into the arena, the gates were thrown open for the bull to come into view. This bull must have been the great-grandsire of Ferdinand, for he peered into the ring rather coyly, and with graceful hesitation, took several steps forward. Then most unexpectedly, he turned tail, jumped over the fence that protects the spectators from the spectacle, and ambled contentedly among the scurrying crowds. With the help of a dozen men the bull was corralled and once more forced into the ring. Now they pelted him with banderillas (gay rosettes with barbed darts) that burrowed into his hide, but even under this annoyance, he trotted around, trying to show his audience that he was a peaceful and harmless animal. This exasperated his tormentors, who began systematically to heap upon him every variety of abuse. Ferdinand himself could not have been more patient, but the time came when snorting and tossing his head in the air, he lunged at the matador, and with one horn, ripped his scalp wide open.

I had wondered how it would affect us to see the bull killed. We loved animals and were becoming more and more in sympathy with the poor beast. As the matador fell, Alice, Sarah and I—all three of us—rose from our seats, clapping our hands, and yelled, "Hurray!"

Mother spoke quickly and firmly, "It is time to go!" and we followed her. She explained, "I was sure you did not want to see the bull killed, and if we had stayed and made such an exhibit of our feelings, we might not have been able to get away."

Biskra had a lure for us that European places lacked. Every

day long trains of camels came either trekking in, or trekking out. Some of the caravans were going out heavily loaded with goods to be distributed in other desert towns. Other caravans were coming in, with the camels loaded with dates. All the caravans halted at the watering trough, at the outskirts of the town, and here we loved to go to watch that continuous, strange panorama—Oriental women mounted on camels; half-naked children investigating everything; camels making strange, weird noises, getting up and lying down, making funny faces, or placidly chewing. Whenever there was a lull after lunch or breakfast, some one would propose, "Let's go to the watering trough," and that meant go and stay till we had to return for another meal. In Biskra it was also absorbingly interesting to watch the trains arrive, sit on the veranda of the hotel, or walk in the Garden of Allah and meet the various races of people. The simple daily routine offered so much diversion in this desert town that by night we were more than ready to retire.

Whenever we had been asked by the Arab guides for the privilege of taking us to see the native dances, we had always flatly refused until the wife of the manager of the hotel begged us to go in order to help out their Arab guide, who was a nice sort of fellow with a family to support, and who recently had had very little to do. We agreed to let him take us the following night. Although we were anxious to start right after dinner, he insisted that to see the dances we must wait until dark.

It was almost nine o'clock when we finally set out. Sarah and Alice walked with the guide, and Mother and I followed. We stopped to greet some gayly arrayed young women from Tougourt, an oasis further south. They had come to Biskra to become prostitutes till they had earned enough money to return home, marry, and live happily ever afterward. They wore their gold pieces hanging in chains looped about their heads, and under the chin. Ankles, as well as arms, were heavy with bracelets. Fingernails and toenails were deeply stained with henna.

As we were sauntering along, several times a man had seemed to push us to one side, but as the streets were full of people, I did not allow myself to think it meant anything until the guide led us into a very narrow street, so narrow that one could span it with arms extended. When we reached the middle of this street, someone clutched the neck of the guide and pinned him against the wall. Waiting for nothing more, and seizing Mother and Sarah by the hand, Alice, too, having firm hold of Sarah, I rushed madly with them through that passageway, stumbling and pushing rudely past every one we met. I expected to find that the little street ended in a fonduk (a place for herding camels), but instead, it opened on a wide street that I immediately recognized, and that enabled me to find the way quickly back to the hotel.

Soon the Arab guide came to explain that the man who had attacked him was jealous, and that no harm would have come to us. His tale did not seem to satisfy either the manager of the hotel or his wife, who begged us to leave Biskra the next morning. They related a tale of a similar attack on a man and his wife, and confessed that they did not trust the Arabs and much preferred us to leave before anything regrettable happened.

Landing at Marseilles on the return trip, we went to Geneva, Switzerland, and from there to Berne. I was anxious to see the work of Herr Professor Kocher, the great Swiss goiter specialist. He was extremely courteous, and welcomed me every day to his clinic. His large classes of medical students he always addressed in German; to patients he spoke in Swiss; when he talked with the nurse handling instruments, he used only French; but while with me he used a beautiful English, better than I use or hear in the United States.

Every morning he removed from three to six goiters, giving only a local anesthetic, and after the goiter had been removed, he pushed the patient to one side for a half hour or more before tying the vessels and completing the operation.

Herr Professor Kocher invited me to dine at his home, where I could meet his wife and the son who now, since his father's death, has taken his place. His wife, a hospitable, gracious lady, did all of his writing and knew everything that he was doing. I was interested in observing that the maid who waited on the table wore spotless white cotton gloves. I have never seen this custom in any other private home, but it pleased me greatly, and gave a sense of asepsis in the handling of food.

From Berne we went to Berlin where I observed an unusual course in military surgery. Two years before in the Mayo Clinic, I had met Professor Schmieden, now an assistant to Herr Professor Biers, who was giving a course in military surgery. No women, not even nurses, were allowed in the operating room, and when I heard that, I was most anxious to attend at least one clinic. Dr. Rosa Engelman, who had been on the Board of Health in Chicago, and to whom I had always referred all sick children, was browsing around among the clinics in Berlin. We joined forces and begged Dr. Schmieden to get permission for us to attend these military clinics as observers. He did so, and it really was a course of great value to me.

The outstanding feature of the clinic was to operate with a minimum of supplies and assistance. The naked patient was brought in on the bare metal cart, and Herr Professor Biers, in his uniform with coat removed, but without sterile gown for himself or sheets for the patient, performed the operation without assistance, using only a knife, a needle, a couple of hemostatic forceps, two sutures, a package of sterile gauze sponges and two sterile towels. Each step of the operation was done with care and precision. In lieu of retractors, the tissues were sutured to expose the field of operation. This surgery seemed like that of William Mayo, who always had little assistance and was constantly cutting from his technique everything not an absolute necessity. Such courses furnish not only good military training, but intrinsic surgical training as well.

From Germany we went on to France for a brief stay in Paris. We saw all of the sights that were starred in our Baedeker, but my memory of the Louvre is not of rare and wonderful pictures. Instead I recall most vividly its toilet: a very large empty room with a stone floor slanting to the center where there was an exit for the water that flowed continuously over its sloping sides.

Here the visitors squatted at random. The picture of well-dressed women publicly sitting on their heels with their clothing twisted around their waists can never be forgotten by anyone who has attended such an exhibition. I approve of the squatting position for defecation and consider it a preventive for constipation, but it was the publicity that disturbed me.

Another surprise was to find in all of the Paris hotels, as part of the bathroom furniture, funny little seats quite apart from the toilet seat and designed for taking vaginal douches. Since I looked upon vaginal douches as the cause of many leucorrheas, I was glad that France was the only country where I ever saw such provisions.

I was glad to leave France, and after a look at the Brussels exposition, we went to London, where we stayed for a month before sailing for home. In London I met a woman surgeon as skillful as Herr Professor Kocher—Dr. Aldrich Blake, who a few years after I left London, was made Dame Aldrich Blake. In 1910 she was operating at the New Hospital for Women, and morning after morning, I attended her surgical clinics. There were other women surgeons and prominent women physicians in London, but I could never bear to miss a morning with Dame Aldrich Blake, and saw no one else's work. Before I visited London again, she had died, and her public memorial was the only reminder of her superb surgical achievements.

When we returned, we sailed from Southampton, England, where we bought strawberries that in size were more like large plums or apricots than berries. Sarah and I stayed in our upper berths during the entire voyage and when we appeared to greet the Goddess of Liberty, our fellow-passengers took us for stowaways. We were not seasick, but we were conversation-sick and preferred to read or sleep the time away.

It was difficult to believe that a year in foreign countries could so enhance our love for our own land that Sarah would weep when she looked at the big engines in the New York Central Station, or that Alice and I would stop to stare admiringly at men and women on the street.

15

COOK COUNTY HOSPITAL

VERY SOON after my return from Europe I received my third invitation to become a member of the staff of the Women and Children's Hospital, and I accepted.

After attending two staff meetings I discovered that: the trustees had little interest except in the finances; the board of lady managers were using the hospital as a social outlet; and the matron, functioning as a superintendent, was catering to the lady managers and serving neither the hospital nor the staff.

I voiced my disapproval of conditions too loudly, too publicly, and too positively, and in consequence, was called to a Star Chamber session with the ladies. What I had left unsaid I now emphasized and was not surprised or regretful when my resignation was demanded. Dr. Lindsay Wynekoop and Dr. Harriet Barringer Alexander, my staunch supporters, suffered the same fate.

A few months after this debacle we learned that the trustees, with a view to settling their troubles once and for all, were negotiating a deal to sell the hospital property and with the proceeds endow a Mary Thompson ward in the Presbyterian Hospital of Chicago.

Dr. Wynekoop, Dr. Alexander and I met the trustees and demanded: first, the resignation of all of the men on the board of trustees, all of the lady managers and the matron; second, the appointment of a board of all women trustees and a staff of women physicians to whom the management of the hospital should be intrusted. On our own initiative and without authorization from anyone we promised that if the staff were given control, it would be responsible for any deficit that might occur, and would liquidate the $6,000 deficit then existing.

The trustees would not consider turning over the hospital to our management just on our promise, but insisted on our securing backers. We finally succeeded in getting them to name the amount of $10,000 as the sum for which to seek a sponsor.

Although we had only a mere handful of wealthy friends and patients, with dogged determination to meet the demands of the trustees, I talked our dilemma over with the late Mr. J. W. Stevens, builder of the Stevens Hotel. He rose to the occasion and wrote the following letter:

> To whom it may concern:
> I do not know any of the women physicians connected with the Women and Children's Hospital, but I know Dr. Bertha Van Hoosen and will be responsible for any indebtedness that she may see fit to incur.

To this blanket bargain he signed his name. To me it was like a parliamentary vote of confidence, but, when I proudly presented it to the trustees, they received it as so much waste paper. They did not want one man as guarantor, but a group or body of individuals.

In answer to this demand, we obtained the sponsorship of the members of the Chicago Woman's Club, who not only offered their support but also elected two of their members to report to the trustees. In a subsequent meeting the trustees told the women that what they wanted was not promises but a trust fund to secure them against deficits. At this point Ella Flagg Young offered to assume the responsibility of the trust fund. I appreciated her loyalty but thought that the women doctors themselves should shoulder the burden. Confident that they would not disappoint me, I telephoned each one of nineteen outstanding women physicians to come at nine the next morning to the First National Bank with $500 to be left in escrow as her share of the trust fund. There was not a quitter or a niggard among them. They all came and by noon the trust fund had been completed, and the new staff took over the management of the hospital. A group of superior women were appointed to fill the many vacancies on the board of trustees and a Cook County trained nurse was installed as superintendent.

Our personnel could not have been improved, but the hospital itself, its furnishings and equipment were discouraging. The cement floors were crumbling and full of holes. The kitchen range was so old that cook after cook refused to stay. The last one gave just one look, saying, "Who in hell can cook on that!" and left. There was so little linen and china that pillow cases were used in lieu of towels, and drinking glasses for tea and coffee. There were no diet kitchens and only one immense operating room. All the beds were low (about a foot high)—not a regular hospital bed in the building. The hospital had never been electrified but was lighted with gas. Even worse than the ramshackle equipment was the din and clatter of the two streetcars that crossed and ran, one in front of, and the other behind the hospital.

To incur no new deficit and to pay off the old, meant that we must have the hospital well filled with paying patients every day. My own finances have never worried me as much as did those of the hospital for the next three years. I was determined to have no deficit. Yet, one month, what I had dreaded happened. There was a deficit of $300! Fearful of the effect this might have upon the nineteen trust-fund contributors, I told the superintendent that I had just received an anonymous gift of $300 to endow a bed for the Trade Union girls, and gave her a check for that amount. It did not fool the superintendent, but it hoodwinked everyone else.

At the end of three years not only was there no indebtedness, but the hospital had been thoroughly reconditioned and electrified from the kitchen to the operating room. We had received some endowments and the hospital was making money. The trustees now assumed responsibility and returned to each doctor her share of the trust fund.

The Women and Children's Hospital was now a going concern, and I felt as much its founder as modest Mary Thompson ever did. As a member of its staff I had every opportunity to care for my private and dispensary patients. I had no teaching position and no clinic, except the dispensary clinic in connection with the hospital. I had never been better situated, mentally or economically, to take on a big job and, surprisingly enough, the job appeared.

To teach operative surgery had long been my cherished ambition and when I learned that, for the first time, the Civil Service Board of Cook County was to hold competitive examinations for positions on the gynecological staff of the Cook County Hospital, I was tempted to enter the contest and compete with my colleagues. I had received many college credits without taking examinations; all my residencies had been by appointment—even my licensure to practice was obtained by endorsement and not by a state board examination. In consequence, I was curious to see what kind of showing I could make on paper. Perhaps, if I had known that all the marks of the contestants would be posted on the central pillar of the City Hall, I would not have had sufficient self-confidence to register as an applicant for the examination.

In 1898 I had hesitated and finally refused to accept the position of Chief of Staff of the Women and Children's Hospital. Now, in 1913, just fifteen years later, I was eager to get a position that would mean operating an entire morning two or three times a week on patients who were too poor ever to become, or to send me, private paying patients. The true spirit of teaching had taken possession of me. As love, not money, makes marriage successful, so it is with teaching.

Three hundred men physicians took the examinations offered by the Civil Service Board. I was the only woman physician. That I might make first place, which would entitle me to become head of the gynecological staff, had never occurred to me, and came as a total surprise. I refused to believe the good news until I had actually received the official card with my grade and notification to begin my service on the first Monday in September, 1913.

Soon after my notification, one of the newly-appointed associates came to my office with the information that the civil service examiners had made a mistake in marking our papers and that another physician, not I, had really made first place. I did not scream or pound the floor with my heels, but I felt just like a baby from whom the dog has snatched a piece of candy.

The visitor stressed, "You know the doctor who made first place is a foreigner, and I am sure you would not wish him to be treated unfairly."

Then he proceeded, "There are a number of plans. All who have taken the examination might resign and take another examination; or petition the Civil Service Board to give the foreign-born man who made first grade, his rightful place; or you, who made first place, could proffer him yours, and step down to the position of associate." To every remark and every plan that he brought forward, I repeated over and over, "I will go over to the civil service rooms."

Time after time he reiterated, "It would be of no use to go to the civil service rooms, for the Board has already placed this physician on the eligible list; I am sure they will do no more unless great pressure is made, but as he is a foreigner, we should see that justice is done."

The interceding associate physician remained an hour with me, but I could find nothing I dared trust myself to say except, "I will go to the Civil Service Board." I was glad to see him depart, and when I reached home, I cried. I could not eat. Alice advised me to put it out of my mind—that I had my appointment, and should pay no attention to these doctors.

All night my mind seethed and swirled in rapid cerebration. In the morning I went to the Women and Children's Hospital, ten miles away, and after seeing my patients, started for home, returning by the long route through Douglas Park, in order to get hold of myself and make a more agreeable companion for dinner. Western Avenue was bleak and lonely, and while riding between vacant lots and open spaces, I reached such a state of morbid depression that I actually heard a voice say, "He is a foreigner."

As though a flash of lightning had illuminated the recesses of my brain, all was clear. I knew now what I was going to do. I stepped up the tortoise-like speed of my electric automobile, and when I arrived home, rushed into the house and telephoned a member of the Cook County Civil Service Board. I explained, "I understand that I did not make first place, that there was a mistake in marking the examination papers, and that first place has been made by another physician. May I ask that the naturalization papers of this physician be verified?"

The sympathetic reply was, "It's just too bad for those doctors to worry you; they have gone over examination papers at the civil service rooms and made so much trouble that everyone has been annoyed with them. Don't pay the slightest attention to anything they say—but as to the naturalization papers, I am sure that they always receive more attention than the scientific papers; it's very doubtful that a mistake has been made. Nevertheless, since you request it, the naturalization papers of all foreigners who took the examination shall be reinspected."

I heard no more of this mistake until a month later when I was looking over interns' papers with Dr. Stowe, who remarked, "They are going to increase the number on the gynecological staff, and I am going on service with you in the fall."

"Why," I said, "what about the doctor who was placed first on the eligible list because the Civil Service Board had made a mistake as to his marks?"

"I guess you know," and he seemed to think I did.

"I know nothing," I said.

"He and two others did not have naturalization papers."

"Oh, you voices," I whispered.

"What did you say?" inquired Dr. Stowe.

"This is a good paper," I muttered.

When I went to the Cook County Hospital to begin my service on the first Monday in September, if I had been sure that there had been a mistake in looking over the naturalization papers and not in marking the examination papers, I would not have entered the warden's office with agitation and a distressing inferiority complex. Not knowing, I waited anxiously three quarters of an hour without receiving any attention, although the warden saw many who had come long after I did. I finally approached his desk, and timidly asked if I could be shown to the women's surgical ward. He looked at me fiercely. "Who are you?" he growled.

I replied, "Dr. Van Hoosen."

He roared, "Well, if you have come here with a chip on your shoulder, you are in the wrong pew!"

I did not warn him that I had a whole woodpile on my shoulder, but stunned by such an unprovoked assault, I spoke up sharply, "I came to work—show me the women's ward!"

At that he called the resident physician, who graciously conducted me to the intern on service. The intern seemed delighted and informed me, "One of the staff physicians came early this morning and divided up the patients. We have two for you to operate on this morning. The first is a large ovarian tumor."

I was surprised and a little relieved. "I think I would like to examine the first case."

The intern led the way toward the preparation room, saying to my astonishment, "Oh, that's unnecessary; she is all prepared, with sterile drapes and everything."

I had never operated on a patient without making an examination, even if superficial, and though I did not want to appear a fussy woman, I was determined to diagnose the case myself.

"I am sorry; I know I seem unreasonable, but drapes or no drapes, I must examine the patient."

He smiled. "All right, you may," he agreed.

I inspected the case and found that instead of an ovarian tumor, the woman was pregnant, full term. In my dilemma, I implored the intern, "Please call the doctor who said this was an ovarian tumor. I want to see him in consultation."

The doctor came, and after passing his hand lightly over the enlarged abdomen, volunteered, "Why, we have an ovarian tumor."

At this my tension broke, and I almost shouted. "Take the patient away—I never want to see her again!"

The astonished men followed me, and without further conversation, I repaired to the operating room and began to scrub for the second operation assigned me. When I had cooled off, I returned to the ward and listened to the regular heartbeat of the "ovarian tumor."

"Listen!" I offered the stethoscope to the intern.

He laughed, "Oh yes, we are all agreed that it's a baby, and not a tumor."

If, in my first case, I had made such a stupid, careless mistake as to operate for a tumor and find a pregnancy, I should not have been able to outlive the damning deed. This experience taught me that henceforth I must walk gingerly.

Many years passed happily for me in the tremendous service of this more than two-thousand-bed County Hospital before another incident, the analogue of my first harrowing experience, occurred. The occasion was the annual meeting of the American College of Surgeons. It was held in Chicago, and Dr. Mary McLean of St. Louis attended as my guest. I secured tickets for her to one of the clinics at Cook County Hospital. After the clinic I met her and asked, "How did the morning go? Cook County Hospital always has something rare to show."

She closed her lips tightly, and spoke in a low voice, "Don't mention it. I cannot talk about it."

My interest was whetted because the operator had been the doctor with whom I had had my first skirmish in connection with the "ovarian tumor" ten years before.

The next day, goaded by curiosity, I saw one of the nurses who had been present at the "unmentionable" clinic. I began, "Well, I hear you had a great time yesterday."

189

Then the nurse, without further urging, poured out the story. "Wasn't it terrific? Before the operation the interns told the doctor that that patient, instead of having a fibroid tumor, might be pregnant, but nothing stopped him. I went into the operating room just as the uterus was laid in a big basin. The junior intern turned the specimen over, and out rolled the baby. You know I am a Catholic, and seizing a bottle of holy water I baptized the baby."

I gasped, "You baptized that baby before all those visiting doctors?"

"Why, yes, of course; I am a Catholic."

The mills of God grind slowly. . . .

Cook County Hospital, in Chicago, like all large eleemosynary medical institutions, furnishes material for clinical instruction in every branch of medicine.

Since surgery, with its many technically intricate major operations, is the most difficult to teach of all branches of clinical medicine, an opportunity to serve on the Cook County Hospital Gynecological Staff was tremendous, for here not only could I have access to a superabundance of surgical material, but my surgical pupils would be the successful candidates in a competitive examination for Cook County internships, in which all Chicago medical schools participated.

After my first year in service I discovered I was especially fortunate in being first choice of the interns. It had long been the custom for the interns to choose their attending men, the choice given them in the order of their examination grades. In this way I had the pleasure of teaching the cream of the interns.

On the surgical service the interns served three months as junior and three as senior. During the junior service I saw to it that the intern learned the steps of my operative technique, recognition of body tissues, the role of assistant, and familiarization with surgical instruments and materials. In the senior, I allowed the intern to perform parts of each operation, beginning with the simplest and proceeding to the most difficult, until an entire operation could be entrusted to the senior intern, with the assistance of his junior.

In teaching surgery by this practical progressive system, I became proficient in properly evaluating surgical difficulties, in seeing my own operative procedures in slow-motion performance, in curbing the reckless and intrepid one, and encouraging the timid and hyper-conscientious.

During my thirteen years' service in this big county hospital I had the satisfaction, as an intimate responsible guide, of conducting more than three score young men into the exacting field of surgery.

The inferiority complex that took possession of these unusually equipped Cook County interns just before their services ended, when they were faced with beginning private practice, can be understood only by realizing that association with a top-ranking staff had increased the interns' professional standards more rapidly than the interns' service had increased their scientific standards. Long after midnight the Cook County intern might be found writing up histories or making laboratory tests.

One day I said to Dr. Frederick Tice, the dean of staff members, "What motivates these boys? They work too hard, yet no one puts any pressure on them."

Dr. Tice, with a faraway look, as though scanning his own Cook County internship, answered slowly, "It is tradition."

In this big municipal hospital, for thirteen years I mingled with the members of the staff (all men), the interns, nurses and patients and knew no differences created by sex. When I entered those wide doors that were never closed against a public made up of all races, colors and religions, sex, like a cloak, was cast aside. Never have I felt such freedom, even in a hospital staffed by women. Here was no money—the staff and interns worked harder than I had ever seen doctors work, but without pay, and the patients paid nothing for the services they received. Here was no color line to offend—black and white lay side by side in the same ward and all were treated alike.

At first it was hard to get used to, and when my intern, a young man with perfect social training, pointing to the door of his room, said, "Oh, by the way, if ever you feel tired and want to rest or take a nap just use my room as if it were your own," I thanked him, but shuddered at the stir it would make if I were caught fast asleep, like Goldilocks, on my intern's bed. Several years later I laughingly told another intern about this gentlemanly offer. He looked at me with eyes wide open like a four year old's and said, "You don't know us interns. Why, you could go into any man's room, and do anything you cared to, and if some fellow should criticize you we would take him into the alley and beat him to a jelly."

At the Cook County Hospital I always began operating promptly at eight o'clock three mornings in the week, and in order that it should be sharp eight instead of eight-thirty, I arrived at the hospital early enough to eat breakfast with the intern on service, always a gracious person, who never failed to join me in the dining room. In this way I came to know socially this wonderful group of medical men.

One of my interns, Dr. Moorehead, whose father was chief of the surgical staff in Mercy Hospital, had been educated for the Jesuit priesthood until he was within one year of graduation. One of his theological classmates, Reverend Patrick Mahan, S.J., often had breakfast with us.

This rather intimate acquaintance resulted in an invitation, in 1918, for me to serve as Acting Head and Professor of Obstetrics in the Loyola University Medical School, where Dr. Moorehead had become Acting Dean, and Father Mahan, Regent of the school.

16

HEAD OF OBSTETRICS

I KNEW that no woman in the world had ever held the position of Head and Professor of Obstetrics in a coeducational medical school. I was at the same time keenly aware that the obstetrical department of Loyola was an Old Mother Hubbard's cupboard —bare, like the Women and Children's Hospital when we took it over in 1911.

Nevertheless, I was not filled with fear or hesitation. As a child I had created Christmas presents, year after year, out of mere nothings. I had taught calisthenics, anatomy, and embryology when each week I was cramming to learn enough to teach the next. My most recent experience had been to bring a hospital from a condition of decay to a state of order. However, I did not underestimate my job.

This teaching position, Head and Professor of Obstetrics in the Loyola University School of Medicine, of all my teaching ventures, was the greatest tax upon my energy and resources, and I do not minimize the teaching that I did in the University of Illinois College of Medicine, where I gave weekly surgical clinics, summer and winter, for eight years. The outstanding difference between the work I did in the University of Illinois College of Medicine, and that in the Loyola University School of Medicine was that in the former I, alone, was responsible for the clinical material, the operations and the lectures, while in the latter, I was responsible for each one of the fifteen teachers in my department.

These unpaid teachers depended for their support on their private obstetrical practices. Consequently, there were many absences for which substitute teachers had to be notified to be on hand at a moment's notice, to teach first one subject, then another, without a clear idea of what the student had already assimilated.

Moreover, all these teachers were expected to be enthusiastic and eager to bestow time, energy and money on their teaching, and in addition, to do research and create without looking forward to a visible reward. If the head of the department could have had salaried positions, or positions with opportunity for advancement, to offer these teachers, the problem would have been easier to solve. If the head of the department herself could have been a full-time salaried teacher, this too, would have been very advantageous.

During my first year as Acting Head of the Department of Obstetrics in Loyola University School of Medicine before it received its A grade, there was a very large class of seniors, numbering around two hundred, none of whom had ever seen a confinement case, much less assisted in a birth. Half of the class was to graduate in the coming March, and the other half in June.

In three months I had the task of providing opportunities for one hundred medical students to see twelve deliveries apiece. Fortunately, I had control of the obstetrical department in the Women and Children's Hospital of Chicago, where we were delivering all the patients under twilight sleep. This made it possible for me to have a section of eight or ten men students present at every delivery, for which, whether day or night, they were telephoned. The details and complications in this arrangement presented heroic obstacles. However, when March came, each student had seen twelve deliveries, the number required at that time by the State Board for graduation.

This method was followed for two years, at the end of which

time I resigned from the Women and Children's Hospital. This resignation improved rather than frustrated my teaching facilities, for it left me free to accept a position on the staff of the Frances Willard Hospital, which was located next door to the Loyola University Medical School. The medical school had a contract with this hospital whereby the school paid for a ward of clinical patients and, on the other hand, the heads of departments in the school, if they desired, could become members of the hospital staff without payment of the usual fee of five hundred dollars.

I had long wished to take advantage of this hospital teaching contract, but felt that if I should resign from the Women and Children's Hospital it would be like desertion. Then too, the medical school paid the Women's hospital more than a thousand dollars a year for the right to send their students there for observing deliveries.

I did not have to decide this, for according to my slogan, "Every hour brings light," the decision came without my making an effort. For almost ten years I had thrown into the Women and Children's Hospital every ounce of my mental and physical energy, yet I am sure that my "pernicious activity," to quote a staff colleague, had made me at times a disturber of the peace, a thorn in somebody's flesh. The superintendent's high regard and affection for me also helped to arouse suspicions on the part of some, that she was partial to me.

This superintendent, a German and a Cook County trained nurse, seemed to me to be omnipresent, omniscient and omnipotent. I discovered one day that she knew what medicine and the exact dose of it that every patient in the hospital was taking. She could balance the books, run the switchboard, manage the operating rooms or, at a moment's notice, cook the meals for the entire hospital family.

Her hands were red, like her plain face, but to me she was beautiful—a symbol of hospital efficiency.

I am sure that for years the trustees had borne patiently with me, with the superintendent, my patients and my medical students, but the time had come when the hospital had a bank balance of over $150,000 instead of a deficit, and could get along without us.

About this time I was informed that the superintendent would have to reform, stay in her office and see people from there. At first I thought it a joke, a funny kind of compliment. Then she was caught red-handed hanging curtains, and was discharged.

My turn came soon after the superintendent's dismissal. The first step was effected by a rule barring all cancer patients from entrance into the hospital. I had been doing some cancer research, and had cured one patient of widespread and advanced cancer. The next step was to exclude from the hospital all male medical students. Finally the trustees made a rule that every doctor should pay for any meal eaten in the hospital dining room. In response to this rule I took my lunch to the hospital and ate it out of a tin dinner pail while I sat in a conspicuous place on some window sill.

When the trustees asked me to resign I felt like a young girl in the beautiful square dances of the Nineties, when she leaves the arms of one partner to fall into the embrace of another. Without a feeling of resentment I left the Women and Children's Hospital, where I had shouldered such heavy financial and professional responsibilities, to become the only woman member on the staff of the Frances Willard Hospital, with its intriguing amphitheater.

Unfortunately, although it helped me greatly in teaching practical obstetrics to have an amphitheater that would seat a hundred students, there were other problems to solve. The Willard Hospital had no free service, and I had to raise the money for clinical cases, or pay for them out of my own pocket.

In 1920 I was appointed to the obstetrical service of the Cook County Hospital where I gave time instead of money, for only staff members were allowed to demonstrate deliveries to medical students. Long hours and many nights were spent in this practical teaching.

When the medical school became affiliated with four Catholic hospitals, arrangements were made for students to go in residence for a week, to see from twenty-five to fifty deliveries. The last few years the school has been affiliated also with the Maternity Center, where students receive two weeks' training in the outpatient department, delivering patients themselves.

Besides developing opportunities for student practice in delivering babies, I made an effort to institute courses of manikin practice, to collect pathological material for microscopic study of diseases of the pregnant woman, to develop prenatal clinics, to secure motion pictures showing pathological deliveries, normal deliveries, and even birth in animals. It would have been impossible to bring the obstetrical department up to an A standard, considering our limited facilities, had not the dean and the regent stood by me.

For many years I had hoped to be instrumental in creating a big maternity hospital for the middle-class working people, where a woman for a fifty-dollar flat rate could be delivered and given ten days' care, while at the same time her young children could be kept in an adjoining creche, under the same management.

I thought such an institution ought to be in charge of some prominent order of nuns, and directly under the management of the Loyola University School of Medicine. A prenatal clinic for mothers, and a pediatric clinic for their children, would furnish a volume of material for teaching and meet the need of people in moderate circumstances.

Realizing that a Catholic Medical School, under the Catholic Church, had the means to put this over successfully and, at the same time, do something to meet the birth-control problem which was troubling the Church, I visited His Eminence, Cardinal Mundelein, to talk the matter over. He was interested, even enthusiastic, and at once set about to find a man to finance the plan. While I was in Europe two years after this pleasant meeting with the Cardinal, Mr. Lewis of Chicago came forward with the necessary funds to start the project.

The old Lakota Hotel, a fourteen-story structure, well built and located at Thirtieth and Michigan Avenue, was purchased, and when I returned from the Medical Women's International Association meeting in Paris, Father Mahan, Regent of the Loyola University School of Medicine, greeted me with, "Well, you'll be happy to know that your plans are about to be carried out. Mr. Lewis has bought the old Lakota, and Dr. Hanrahan is at work on plans to convert it into a two or three-hundred-bed maternity hospital."

The Lewis Maternity Hospital has been a help in solving the "family" problem for the middle classes, but for the purpose that most interested me, the teaching of obstetrics, it has been a dream unfulfilled. Cardinal Mundelein's veneration for birth would not allow him to give clinical privileges to medical students at the Lewis Memorial Hospital, although one of the necessary requirements for medical students is practical instruction in midwifery.

The president, dean and regent were courageously loyal to me at the time the medical school received its A grade. Quite accidentally, after asking the clerk to get me some blanks, my eye caught a letter on her desk. I knew that I ought not to read it, but at a glance I saw that it was about me, and I not only read it—I reread it.

The letter was from the American Medical Association to the Loyola University School of Medicine, and after stating that their recent survey had resulted in placing the Loyola University School of Medicine among the Grade A schools, they made the suggestion that took my breath, "We recommend that you put a man at the head of the Department of Obstetrics."

I was not prepared for such an exhibition of sex prejudice from the American Medical Association, of which I had been a member for a quarter of a century. However, I did not intend to make Loyola suffer for my sex.

The following day, meeting the dean in the corridor of the Mercy Hospital, I began, "I am so delighted that we have the A grade, but I consider the standing and growth of an institution of learning of so much more importance than the interests of an individual that I would be unhappy to hamper in any way the future of Loyola. More than that, I want you to know that my work with you has been its own reward."

At that the dean inquired, "What are you talking about! You have been appointed Head of Obstetrics, and there is nothing more to discuss. Hasn't Father Fury written you?"

I shook my head.

"He will."

I reported this conversation to Alice, who laughed. "That was a beautiful speech! Now they will feel free to let you out."

A week later Alice asked, "Has Father Fury written you yet?"

I replied, "No."

"All right," she warned, "they will let you down easy."

Another week passed, and Alice slyly suggested, "Got your letter?" I shook my head.

The next day I had a telephone message to meet Father Fury at seven in the evening at St. Ignatius High School.

At exactly seven I arrived at the big bleak building adjoining the church, was ushered into an enormous high-ceilinged, unfurnished room hung with life-sized paintings of Popes and Archbishops, and seated in the only chair. It seemed long before the door opposite me opened, and Father Fury, with a beaming florid face, came with quick short steps across the room and extended his hand. "I am so sorry! You are so busy I should not have intruded on your time—but you must forgive me. It was an old man's weakness. I wanted to tell you face to face that you have been appointed Head of Obstetrics of the Loyola University School of Medicine. We appreciate the splendid work you have done in helping us get an A grade. I know there is prejudice against women, and we are prejudiced too—but it is for you, and not against you."

I did not sink to the floor and clasp his feet, nor did I fall upon his neck and cover it with tears and kisses, but I am sure that with all of those feelings pent up within me I must have seethed like a singing teakettle. His cloth was the only thing that kept the lid on.

17

MEDICAL WOMEN ORGANIZE

IN THE FIFTIES, women's medical schools sprang up like mushrooms all over the country, due to the fact that women were barred from other medical schools. The faculties of these schools were, of necessity, made up of men physicians who were in sympathy with the study of medicine by women.

This situation was responsible for a division of the men in the profession into two groups, one for and the other against medical women.

Dissension between these two groups grew steadily until in the Sixties and Seventies it had reached a point where medical men teaching in women's medical schools, or consulting with women physicians, were threatened with expulsion from their respective state and county societies if they continued in that forbidden practice.

The American Medical Association meeting at San Francisco in 1871 was like a tournament in the days of King Arthur— each man jousting for his lady. Feelings ran so high that it was thought wise to let the subject rest and it did not come up again until 1876 at the Philadelphia meeting. It might not have come up at this time had not an unlooked-for argument presented herself to the Credentials Committee. The State of Illinois had sent as a delegate one Dr. S. H. Stevenson whose credentials were accepted and approved without question. However, when the delegate appeared in the guise of an attractive woman with all the grace and charm of a social leader, the opposition of the males melted, and Dr. Sarah Hackett Stevenson became the first woman member and the first woman delegate of The American Medical Association.

With the American Medical Association taking the lead, all state and county societies, one by one, extended membership to women physicians.

Coincident with this move was the spread of coeducation through our state medical schools and at the same time, the gradual disappearance of all medical schools for women with the exception of the first one established. With the closing of women's medical schools, nothing was left to replace what had served as a de facto organization for medical women.

Medical women have never been more than a five per cent minority group, and for that reason more than any other, organization seemed highly desirable to some of the women physicians.

The first American Medical Association meeting that I attended (Atlantic City, 1904) was a dreary experience, for I met no one whom I knew, and was too timid to make any new acquaintances.

Four years later, at an American Medical Association meeting in Chicago, I helped to initiate the custom of giving a dinner for the visiting women physicians. Every year for the next seven years, a banquet was part of the entertainment during a medical meeting, but any attempt to organize the medical women was quickly denounced as a move toward segregation.

Accordingly, in the fall of 1915, following a celebration of the fiftieth anniversary of the founding of the Women and Children's Hospital of Chicago by Dr. Mary Thompson, I invited a group of women whom I knew to be enthusiastic for organization, to meet me at the Chicago Woman's Club. At that meeting the medical women organized.

The Press and many friends have often hailed me as the

founder of the American Medical Women's Association, and I would be in danger of attributing to it too much importance were I not conscious of the service and devotion of its membership in the building up of the organization.

My absorbing interest in group cooperation puzzles me, for on the farm where the union is still a stranger, and in college where I never held a class office, I was a strong individualist.

The intense feeling against the organization that was exhibited by medical women in all parts of the United States, especially on the Pacific Coast, demanded great loyalty and courage of its members. Condemning petitions were circulated, and the association might have collapsed had it not been that the entrance of the United States into World War I in April, 1917, demonstrated the importance of our organization.

When the Surgeon-General refused to accept the application for army service of any one of the five thousand women physicians in active practice in the United States, a furor was raised, especially on the Pacific Coast. Again a petition was started, this time not against our organization, but against the class and sex discrimination made by the Surgeon-General. When the huge petition, like a full-term pregnancy, rolled into New York City, it was delivered into the hands of our association for submission to the government. Our future existence was assured.

The women's meetings are held at the same time and same place as those of the American Medical Association, to which all of the members of the American Medical Women's Association also belong. Their work is done through committees.

In 1917, as the first president, I created a War Service Committee and appointed Dr. Rosalie Slaughter Morton as chairman. She occupied that position for one year in which she organized the work and gave the committee the name of American Women's Hospitals. Dr. Crawford of New York City followed Dr. Morton, and in 1919, Dr. Esther Lovejoy, at that time Head of the Public Health Service in Portland, Oregon, took over the chairmanship and has held it ever since.

The American Women's Hospitals has functioned for the past

twenty-nine years, and during that time has sent overseas more than three hundred medical women for active duty in war and postwar relief, and has established more than one hundred hospitals and dispensaries in France, Greece, Serbia and the Near East.

Besides the overseas work, a small maternity hospital has been equipped and maintained in our own Blue Ridge and Cumberland Mountains where conditions demanded relief.

From Tokyo, Japan, after the earthquake in 1923, I cabled Dr. Lovejoy for assistance on behalf of the Japanese women physicians and she answered immediately with the sum of $10,000 to use for the relief of suffering women and children.

During World War II, the American Women's Hospitals cabled either $500 or $1,000 every month to the medical women in each of the countries of Great Britain, Russia, China, and France as long as she was one of the allies. In summarizing the work of the American Women's Hospitals it can be stated that since its creation the committee has collected and expended for war relief an average of $400 every day.

To help financially embarrassed women medical students in whatever school they may be studying, a Scholarship Loan Fund has succeeded in collecting about $30,000, which is constantly circulating.

The chairman of the Committee on History, the late Dr. Kate Campbell Mead, published a history of medical women up to the nineteenth century, and at her death in December, 1941, she had ready for publication a continuation of her first book.

A Library Committee, in charge of a collection known as the Medical Women's Library, is at present organizing a campaign to raise $500,000 with which to erect a building to house their historical material and create a memorial for pioneer medical women.

The Medical Women's Library of the American Medical Women's Association took form in 1933 as an exhibit in the Hall of Social Science of the Century of Progress, Chicago. This exhibit consists of books written by or about medical women;

scrap books with press notices relating to medical, dental and allied science women; and portraits, including paintings in oil, etchings, and photographs of distinguished women in the field of science, both in this country and abroad.

This material that I had been many years collecting was put into exhibit form through the funds of the Medical, Dental, and Allied Science Women's Association, a group functioning exclusively for the duration of the Fair. At the close of the Century of Progress, I presented the exhibit to the American Medical Women's Association through its president, Dr. Lena Sadler, who had contributed much in time, money and service to its creation. Through the kindly offices of Dean D. J. Davis, of the Medical School of the University of Illinois, suitable accommodations have been provided in the Quine Library in Chicago for its housing, with ample stacks for its books and wall space for its pictures.

One of the unique features of this collection is the part concerning distinguished sons and daughters of medical women. The roll of these outstanding names is a long one. The purpose of this collection is to draw the attention to, and perhaps give an irrefutable argument in favor of marriage for medical women.

At the end of a Medical Women's Library leaflet published a few years ago was a paragraph which now appears to have been a horoscope for the library because it foretold the building of a library, plans for which are now being made.

The Committee on Opportunities for Medical Women communicates every year with all the hospitals in the United States that do not admit women interns, in the hope of removing the sex discrimination that bars medical women students from five-sixths of the six hundred hospitals approved for internships. This ban on women interns might be lifted at once if the American Medical Association would make the acceptance of women interns one of the qualifications for hospital approval for interns.

The most outstanding piece of work of the Association was recently accomplished by the Legislative Committee. During the chairmanship and under the instigation of Dr. Emily Barringer of New York, after a tense Congressional hearing, the Sparkman bill, asking for Army and Navy service for women on the same conditions as given to men, was passed, and on April 17, 1942, President Roosevelt signed the bill, making it law. After twenty-five years of persistent effort on the part of the American Medical Women's Association, medical women have been able to join the Army and Navy Medical Reserve Corps.

I cheerfully confess that organized medical women have not only fought for the welfare of the group, but in their own ranks have encountered many differences of opinion.

Now and then we had discussions so full of vigor, if not of venom, that Alice would ask on my coming home after a meeting, "Well, are you returning victorious, or licking your wounds?"

A highlight in the history of the American Medical Women's Association, the first organization of medical women, is its part in organizing the medical women of foreign countries.

At the close of World War I the Young Women's Christian Association found that it had some money remaining in its treasury out of the funds that were to have been devoted to war relief. Realizing the potency of a world convention of distinguished women, and prompted by the interests of peace and Christianity, it invited many foreign women to New York as its guests.

During this conference, a unit of the American Women's Hospitals, just returned to New York City, was given a dinner to which some of the visiting foreign women physicians were invited. It was at this meeting that the International Medical Women's Association was born.

International associations have many advantages over those of only national scope. Foremost is the opportunity for travel. To attend my first international convention in Budapest, in 1909, I took a year off and visited nearly all of the countries in Europe and some in Africa.

My second international convention, in 1929, took me to

Paris. Since our previous European trip did not include Spain, Portugal, and the large cities on the west coast of Italy, we were routed through those countries, and booked to sail from New York City on a Spanish liner, Alfonso XIII.

The evening of the fourteenth of February, when all the lights made the harbor gay, we sailed hopefully away from pie, doughnuts, ice water and hot baths. The next morning the ocean was very rough and became rougher every hour, until by the third day it was absolutely terrifying and continued so through the fourth and fifth. However, the last three days of the journey were calm enough to enable us to crawl out of our berths, where we had been pitched from side to side, day and night for five days, until we were black and blue. When we saw the condition of the furniture and heard the tales of our fellow passengers who had suffered cuts and broken bones, we were thankful to be alive and well. One of the passengers, who was making his twenty-eighth trip across the Atlantic, described the storm as the worst he had ever encountered.

Landing at Vigo, we toured Spain and Portugal, spent a week in Tangier, Morocco, and then sailed from Gibraltar to Italy. We reached Rome the week before Easter.

At my first opportunity I delivered a letter from the regent of the Loyola University School of Medicine, requesting for me an audience with the Pope. The following day I received an invitation on purple stationery, granting the audience with His Holiness, Pope Pius XI, on Holy Monday. The invitation gave directions on how to dress, with a picture of a lady properly garbed for a visit to the Vatican. The manager of our pension, impressed with our invitation, said he would supply the mantillas, a part of the costume. When the day came, we dressed and adjusted our mantillas. Alice was as always, quite correct, but I as usual, was not, for I had on brown shoes, and the directions expressly mentioned black ones. As I looked at them with dismay, I thought of my pair of new, shiny black rubbers, and put them on. Alice laughed, but I could not see why they were any funnier than the mantillas. When we started for the Vatican, the proprietor of the hotel and some of the guests exclaimed, "Why the rubbers?"

"Why not?" I snapped, for I was getting a little touchy on the subject.

It might have been that their query upset me; at any rate, it was I who was responsible for our getting on the wrong car. Alice said it was foolish not to take a taxi from the pension, but I was feeling familiar with Rome and determined to take the streetcar. After a very long ride I made inquiries of the conductor, who looked at us in great amazement, stopped the car, and put us off, but gave no directions. Time was passing, and we were getting nervous. Finally, after running here and there, we got a taxi and said, "Vatican, quick!"

Just as the bell of St. Peter's struck one (the hour for the appointment), we entered between the fancifully dressed Swiss guards, and climbed the longest flight of stairs I have ever seen. And if it had been just one flight! But, no! Flight on flight, until we reached the sixth story, where we were conducted into a room guarded by men dressed in crimson velvet; from there, into another room; and on into a third, which gradually filled with enough people to make a solid row all around the room. Here we stood for three hours, for there were no seats. At four o'clock one of the brocaded-crimson-velvet-uniformed men came in and asked us to kneel. I was nearest to the door and first to be greeted by His Holiness. I kissed his ring and then had an opportunity to watch him as he went to each person. He wore a dress with skirt of white wool reaching the floor, a broad satin belt, a small white skullcap, and white slippers decorated on the toes with diamonds. He was accompanied by the Cardinal who became Pope Pius XII. After the ceremony of kissing the ring, we went into a larger room, where the Pope ascended a platform and blessed those gathered there. As I knelt no one saw my rubbers, and I removed them before my return to the pension, feeling, however, that I had, in living up to directions, shown my appreciation for being allowed to meet such a fine public servant.

We had wanted, on this trip, to buy a piece of wall tapestry, perhaps in Spain, but we found that even Spanish shawls were made in China. We looked in Rome and Naples, but found none. At last, when we reached Florence, we discovered in the Pitti Palace just the tapestries we had been looking for, hanging between the rooms containing that immense art collection. "Let's take one," I suggested, and Alice, as pleased as I, was sure one would not be missed. On leaving the galleries, we went across the street to a little shop, and here at the back of the store we saw a portiere exactly like those that we had coveted in the Pitti Palace, but the storekeeper would not consider selling it.

It was four in the afternoon, and raining, when we returned to Hotel Fiorita. Alice lay down to rest, while I went out to purchase a Roman lamp that I had seen in some shop. I found the shop quite easily, purchased the lamp, and asked the shop-girl, "Where can I buy a portiere like those in the Pitti Palace?"

"If you will wait until Father returns, he can help you," she promised.

He soon came, understood what I wanted, and knew where they might be bought, but insisted on going with me as interpreter. He spoke no English, and I no Italian, but we both knew a little French. Ordering a cab, we visited many stores, but after each failure he would say in French, "My friend has one. I will see him. He may sell it."

As it was getting late, we finally gave up the search and returned to the shop, but to my embarrassment, the kindly gentleman would take nothing for his time or trouble, and his last words as I drove away were, "My friend—"

I found Alice greatly worried and excited. A girl from whom we had bought a linen dress was waiting for her pay, and dinner was ready. I paid the girl, and we went to dinner. Gently and very gradually, I related my experience, but had not yet finished the story when the hotel manager came to say, "There is a gentleman with a flag, waiting to see you."

Not dreaming who it might be, I found my red-haired Italian

friend, not with a flag, but with the Pitti Palace-like portiere, pole and fixtures. The hotel proprietor examined it and said it was very good. I asked the price. With great hesitation he told me that his friend did not feel that he could part with it for less than 700 lire ($35), that his friend valued it very much. When the Fiorita proprietor found that I had only 500 lire with me, he produced the 200 lire and told me to buy it if I wanted it. Whenever I look at that piece of tapestry, I see not just a souvenir of the Pitti Palace, but a lasting tribute to the beauty of the Italian character. I feel and enjoy again that simple, honest, golden-rule treatment accorded me by those two gentlemen of **Florence**.

From Florence we went directly to Paris, to attend the International Medical Women's Association meeting, which was the professional climax to this trip. Nineteen years had passed since the Sixteenth International Congress of Medicine at Budapest when I had experienced that wild and wonderful sensation of reading a paper before foreigners in a strange country—the paper that I read willy-nilly.

I am ashamed to confess that at this meeting in Paris, in an effort to take moving pictures of all the delegates, I missed most of the proceedings of the meetings. For all that, this international congress must have stimulated an appetite for such meetings, for in two years I was planning to attend another.

In 1931, I painted such a rose-colored picture of a vacation trip to the Isthmus of Panama, under the direction of the United Fruit Company, that Alice joined me, and we sailed from New York City in January. The boat was small, one-class, very comfortable, and the cuisine was excellent. I love bananas as much as I do fish and enjoyed having them in some form at each meal. We made a short stop at Jamaica where I resisted my second temptation to buy a string of opals for $100.00. My first had been in Brisbane, Australia.

The medical objective of our trip was the Pan-American Association meeting at Panama, where I read a paper on Corrective

Obstetrics in which I reported fifty cases and described an operation (pubiotomy) whereby a pelvis too small to permit a normal birth is permanently enlarged. This operation is indicated especially in cases of young women who wish to have more than one child, for it not only enables the mother with a narrow pelvis to expel her child normally, but it insures normal deliveries in following pregnancies.

The majority of obstetricians are not surgeons and, for that reason, look upon this operation with disfavor, claiming all manner of mishaps following it, such as a waddling gait, or even inability to walk. They prefer the Caesarean operation, the simplest of all operations, but one that in no way corrects the disability. The late Dr. Frederick Albee of New York City was present when I read my paper. He commented favorably on it and reported cases in which he had performed the operation with great success.

After a week in Panama attending banquets and receptions, we stopped for a few days at Cristobal. Both in Panama and Cristobal we were fortunate in getting reservations in the one hotel which, perfectly appointed and very lovely, was under the management of our Government.

On the return trip we had a week in gay Havana, Cuba, where, for the first time, I learned of a club with a membership running into the thousands, housed in a very large building just opposite our hotel. To me the most interesting thing about this club was that its yearly dues insured its members against any sickness at home or in a hospital. The club was rich and powerful and had been in existence for a long time. Leaving Havana for New Orleans we touched at Guatemala, where the United Fruit Company took all of its passengers on a boat ride up the Sweet River. The boat was a side-wheeler and passed close to the shore, between high, precipitous banks covered with dense jungle growth through which brilliantly colored birds flitted among orchids and other gayer flowers. We arrived at New Orleans in time for the Mardi Gras. This was my third international medical meeting.

Again, five years later, in spite of my apathy in regard to the meeting in Paris, I was overly anxious to attend another meeting of the International Medical Women's Association in Stockholm. This time, not being able to persuade Alice to go, I went with a large group of women physicians from all parts of the United States. We sailed on the good ship Gripsholm that made so many good-will passages during World War II, bringing back to the United States prisoners from all parts of the world.

When I discovered that the Gripsholm had a large swimming pool, I determined to take a swim every morning while on board. Having no bathing suit, I bought three before I found one to suit me. It was all wool, in two pieces, and light green in color. It took up more than its share of room in my suitcase, but no one could have persuaded me not to have taken it. When I announced my intention of swimming every morning, Dr. Ratterman of Cincinnati, the best woman in outdoor sports in the Association, asked if she could join me. In my fetching sea-green suit, covered with a long robe, I descended in the elevator and stepped out onto a platform overlooking the pool. I thought I must be dreaming. I looked at Dr. Ratterman who said, "What are you going to do?" I knew then that it was true—at last the greatest desire of my life had come to pass—everybody, in and out of the pool, except ourselves, was stark naked.

I have often shocked Alice by insisting that I was going to join a nudist colony, and now I could. My answer to Dr. Ratterman's question was, "Look! See!" And I peeled off that heavy, hot, sticky, all-wool suit, and brought it home as a souvenir of what not to wear. On that happy Gripsholm trip to Scandinavia I spent the best part of every morning in the salt-water pool, and enjoyed again the freedom of those first nine months of my life when, naked, I swam in the waters of the womb.

On the way to Stockholm we stopped at Copenhagen and were entertained by the medical women of Denmark. We were guests of an hotel exclusively for women, and every minute of our two-day sojourn was devoted to clinics, visits to institutions, dinners, banquets, luncheons, teas, receptions, and drives. If we had gone for nothing more than the entertainment given by the women doctors in Copenhagen, it would have been well worth the trip across the Atlantic.

In Stockholm, the days were spent in listening to papers and discussions, and the evenings, to attending pompous banquets.

To me, the most important person that I met was the interpreter. She was French and not only interpreted every speech, but actually edited it, so that it came from her lips, fluent and grammatically charming, no matter whether she spoke in English, French or German. Before our next international meeting, she had died. No one since has been able to compare with her in her ability to transform the thoughts of a woman doctor, awkwardly and poorly expressed, into a delightful speech.

In 1937, again without any one of my family, I attended the last meeting of the Medical Women's International Association, which was held in Edinburgh, Scotland. As the women doctors had been entertained in Copenhagen on the way to the Stockholm convention, they were made guests of the London medical women on their way to Edinburgh.

Our opening meeting was held in the University of Edinburgh and we were welcomed by prominent university men. A most beautiful reception took place in the Museum of Fine Arts. I often wonder why our superb public buildings, especially our universities, are not more often used for receptions and conventions.

The programs of these international meetings are unlike those of any other association with which I have ever been connected. There are always two subjects up for discussion and these are chosen at a meeting immediately preceding the one at which the program will be used. Besides the subjects for discussion, three reporters are selected, one for the English speaking countries, one for the French speaking, and one for the German. All members of the association are invited to write a paper on one or both subjects up for study, but are expected to have their papers in the hands of the proper reporter, either English,

French, or German, one year before the date set for the meeting. Each reporter herself, must write a paper based on the abstracted and evaluated papers that have been sent in to her. This paper, too, must be sent to the secretary of the association at least three months before the dated meeting. All of the reporters' papers are printed and ready for distribution when the meeting at which they are to be used is called to order. The reporters speak first on the selected subjects and afterwards they are open for general discussion.

At the Edinburgh meeting I was the English reporter. The work that this position demanded was heavy, for besides papers from the women of Great Britain, her colonies, and the United States, there were papers from Chinese, Japanese, Russian and Indian women. Several European countries used the English language and sent their papers to me. In addition to preparing and sending my paper for publication I had to introduce the subject at the meeting. I also produced and, on my own initiative, showed a visual education film on maternal mortality. This, when set in motion, was automatic and would run for hours without attention. Because of this heavy machine, as well as a large quantity of literature for distribution at the meeting, I embarked in a merchant marine that took nine days to cross the Atlantic but, uniquely, docked in London.

At one of the banquets the usual toast was drunk to the King and Queen. When a decided lull followed, at that moment, I proposed a toast to the Duchess of Windsor. At once there was such confusion and so much rattling of glasses that I thought I had struck the keynote of the evening, but I received so many curtain lectures from my American friends that I am convinced it was a faux pas.

After the convention an opportunity was given us to attend the British Medical Association that is held every two years and to which representatives from all of the colonies come. This year it was held in Belfast, Ireland, and I had the great honor to attend as a foreign guest. I was entertained in the lavish fashion that few people except the English can approach.

In this B.M.A., which corresponds to our A.M.A., I had the feeling that medical women were treated more on a basis of equality and with more natural consideration than they are in the United States. One of Dr. DeLee's films of childbirth was shown and received a splendid ovation. The next B.M.A. was to have been held in South Africa, but the war intervened.

We had four weeks before sailing and spent a few days at the Dublin Horse Show and took an automobile tour through Ireland. Near Cork we spent a night with Trappist monks, whose vows do not permit them to speak. As their guest house was full they gave us beds in the school dormitory, where we and eighteen other occupants slept. Where we slept was of little importance, for we did not get to bed until eleven o'clock and got up at three in order to attend four o'clock mass in the Cathedral hard by. The monks rose at two and were already attending masses when we arrived at four. Between that time and six we heard twenty-seven masses said by different priests at many altars. We were served breakfast in the guest house with the guest monk who was allowed to speak, officiating as host. The slices of bread served us were twelve inches square! Breakfast was enlivened by a bit of excitement over the loss of our one hundred and thirty rosaries that Miss Murray, the only Catholic among the four of us, had handed to one of the priests and asked him to bless. The priest, not understanding English, supposed the rosaries were a gift and did not even open the package.

Our leaving was delayed a couple of hours. Only after vigorous use of the pen and finally employment of sign language, was it possible to locate the lost package. The vows of silence, however holy, are unhandy!

Since we were to sail from Liverpool on our return trip, we made that city our headquarters the rest of the time. This enabled us to visit the Royal Agricultural Show, where I took moving pictures of the stock for Sarah to show her friends in Michigan. We also saw two flower shows, one at Shrewsbury and the other at Southport. To walk through five miles of intensely packed exhibits and see blooms that only England can produce, especially the display of one thousand orchids, is something impossible to forget.

I have attended six international medical meetings, three for women doctors only and three for both men and women. They gave me the same pleasure that I always experience on arriving in the United States after a long sojourn in a foreign country. I love to mingle with people of all nationalities, not of just one. In a foreign country, I tire of the sameness in the population. I miss our happy, handsome, black-skinned people, our smiling, neat Japanese, the burly, black-haired Italians, the well-dressed Jews, the straight-haired Indians with high cheek bones. These international meetings give me just this delightful cosmopolitan feeling, only in an exaggerated form.

It is quite probable that not more than one per cent of the 150,000 doctors in the United States have ever attended an international medical meeting. However, the future promises, that with more sensible international relations and our rapid transportation, these international meetings may be enjoyed by ninety-nine, instead of one per cent of doctors.

18

THE GENUS, HEN MEDIC

MY DUTY toward medical women who desire to become surgeons took definite shape after I had listened to a story about the late Dr. Nicholas Senn. When he became Professor of Surgery in Rush Medical College, then affiliated with the University of Chicago, President Harper asked him, "How many doctors have you trained to take your place? You are a great surgeon, Dr. Senn, but if you have not prepared men to follow in your footsteps and go farther than you have gone, everything you have accomplished is lost."

From that moment I determined to train young women to become surgeons, and measuring by this Harper yardstick, I have trained twenty.

The young women who have spent with me a couple of years or more in surgical training call me "Mother," and I regard them as my "surgical daughters." Like all mothers I have carried them so long close to my heart that I can see no flaws in them, but I try never to omit an opportunity to perfect their technique or increase their knowledge.

On their part they have taught me many things—more than I have imparted to them. Through my work with them, I have learned that there is no such thing as a crystallized, perfect surgical technique, because progress demands constant changes to keep pace with research; that surgical success depends upon an understanding of the natural resistance of the tissues to germs, and this differs in different parts of the body; that the ability of the blood to clot is of more importance than the doctor's skill in catching and tying severed blood vessels; that a limited time of tissue exposure is as important as asepsis, because no permanent asepsis can be maintained outside of an airtight chamber; that constant sponging is a trauma to be avoided except where a clean field is absolutely necessary; that sharp scalpels lessen post-operative pain and promote healing; that surgical violation should be confined to as few tissues as possible; and that all manipulations should be as gentle as though the patient were not anesthetized.

My surgical daughters have convinced me that surgeons should have as prerequisites to their training, courses in the manual arts, such as tailoring, knitting or embroidering, before cutting and sewing the human body. My one assistant who had taken a course in tailoring was able to do the cleverest operating in the shortest time of any woman I have ever trained. Another, Dr. Rose Menendian, who put herself through medical school by embroidering for Marshall Field's in Chicago, is rapidly developing a delightful, bold technique.

One daughter, Dr. Mabel Gardner, had a well established practice in Middletown, Ohio, before she decided to specialize in surgery. Not to interrupt her practice for too long a period, she came to Chicago whenever a vacancy occurred in my service, and filled the position of first assistant. When she had acquired independence, she began to operate in the Middletown General Hospital on her own patients. For a year or two I went to Middletown to assist her with her major operations.

Her first operation was on a woman of seventy who had a huge ovarian tumor. We thought that this would be an excellent case with which to start Dr. Gardner's operating in her home town, for as a rule ovarian tumors are simple to remove. We gave the patient full doses of twilight sleep, and she required no additional anesthetic for the opening of the abdomen and the slow draining off of the contents of the cyst. When the cyst was nearly empty, we removed it, but found behind the cyst a complicating fibroid tumor as large as a five months' pregnancy, and what was more distressing, a cancer filling the cavity of the uterus. After all disease had been removed, we closed the abdomen, and drove to town for a quick lunch. On returning to the hospital, we found the nurse too excited to explain her anxiety. She had left the patient for a second to answer the telephone just outside of the patient's room. As she hung up the receiver, she caught sight of the old lady at the end of the long hall, where she had gone in search of the bathroom. I was so happy that after all we had done to her, she was able to get around without assistance that I kissed everybody and was hungry. The patient lived for many years, proving that her stroll after a major operation hurt no one except the nurse, who almost died of fright. Dr. Gardner soon operated without my assistance, and today is the leading surgeon in that part of the country.

In 1923, as circuit surgeon, I went as far afield as China and operated with some of my surgical daughters in cities from Canton to Peking. My first acquaintance with Chinese women physicians dates from the time that Dr. Mary McLean came to Chicago to get an internship in one of the hospitals for one of her protegees, Dr. Li Yuin Tsao.

I wagered that she would not meet with success and told her, "When you fail, come back, and we will take Li Yuin at the Women and Children's Hospital."

Disappointed and resentful, she returned to accept my offer.

Nevertheless, I began to regret my impulsive bravado and to dread the constant defense of a Chinese intern. I could almost hear such remarks as these: "I won't have a 'Chink' doctor me." "Don't let that foreigner come near me." "Why must we have a foreigner when we haven't enough positions for our own women?"

Quite the reverse. From the moment Dr. Tsao arrived, her tall, handsome, dignified presence was welcomed, and her success was summed up by a small boy who was brought to the hospital for a tonsillectomy. He was given nasty medicine, choked to sleep, and woke up with the worst sore throat that he had ever had. He resented these insults with manly vigor, and kicked, scratched and screamed till he was exhausted. When his aunt came on the following day, he sobbed, "Take me home! Take me home! I hate everybody here, I hate the nurses, I hate the doctors, I hate everybody, 'cept the Chinaman. I love the Chinaman."

Another remarkable Chinese intern followed Dr. Tsao, Dr. Margaret Chung, American-born of Chinese parentage. She never wore Chinese clothes, but on all occasions appeared in a plain black tailored suit, a white silk shirtwaist, and when on the street, a black sailor hat. This costume would have been very inconspicuous had she not always carried a short sport cane.

Dr. Chung had a great aptitude for surgery, and I, as well as others on the staff, gave her unaccustomed opportunities to operate. The first news from her after she began practicing was that she had removed Mary Pickford's tonsils.

In 1938, while I was attending a meeting of the American Medical Women's Association in San Francisco, Dr. Chung sent her big car with its Japanese chauffeur to bring me to her office. The typical and very beautiful Chinese furnishings took my fancy, especially one room, a veritable museum of aeronautic relics and historic pieces which had been contributed by a large and increasing group of flyers, "The Bastards," who call her "Mother Chung." The walls of another room were covered with photographs of motion picture stars who had been her patients.

When I began to operate for out-of-town women M.D.'s in their home-town hospitals, a hospital in the vicinity, or in the home of the patient, I started unconsciously a new kind of practice, and became a circuit surgeon.

In towns small enough to regard the comings and goings of their populace as matter of public interest, the woman M.D. who calls another doctor in her own home town to operate on her patient tacitly acknowledges that he is the better man, and when the patient again needs care, she naturally goes to him. It was to overcome this condition, and to promote the women physicians in small towns within a day's ride from Chicago that I undertook to do their surgical work in their own locality.

In some towns there were good hospitals, in others, poorly equipped ones, or none at all. There were women doctors who did not have a surgical case oftener than every two or three years, while others had many operative cases every month. Occasionally, I went for one operation, but more often I put in six or eight hours operating on from four to six patients each trip. In Muskegon, Michigan, where I operated for Dr. Lunette Powers and the late Dr. Lucy Eames, both of whom had large, general practices, in one day we performed operations on nineteen patients, the last of which we finished at six in the afternoon. This was a limit that I have never since approached except once in Kiukiang, China, where, with Dr. P. Y. Tsao, I did fifteen operations in one day.

I have a record of thirty-six different towns, forty-four hospitals and fifty-eight women physicians on my circuit as itinerant surgeon. Many patients that I operated on have never met me, and do not even know my name. I was to them just another woman who came to help their woman doctor. If it had been otherwise, circuit surgery would have been wasted energy, and have done little or nothing to advance women in medicine.

The most remarkable feature of this circuit surgery was that in no case that I know of did any one of the small town women doctors ever make a mistake in diagnosis. The after-care was entirely in their hands, and here too they stood the test, for in twenty-five years of this variety of surgical practice, we lost only three patients out of the many hundreds of operations performed.

This experience added much to the confidence in, and practice of, small town women physicians, but it was also of untold value to me in developing a foolproof surgical technique, for it was necessary to leave patients in such condition that no trouble would develop after I had departed. All bleeding must be prevented, no septic conditions must arise, the body tissues must not have too much strain put upon them, or the circulation cut off by too many sutures.

Inasmuch as I always found different nurses at every hospital, I carried out a method I had learned at the Mayo Clinic. I used only three kinds of surgical needles: a large, curved cutting needle for the skin, a small, curved round needle for deeper tissues, and a straight cambric needle for the appendix. In the large needle I used silkworm gut; in the small curved one, catgut; and in the cambric one, a linen suture. For abdominal surgery I used number one plain catgut, while in vaginal surgery I used number one chromic catgut. In less than two minutes I could teach the nurse this technique, and in consequence, I did not have to wait for sutures, and never worried or confused the nurse.

It required constant training on my part to use this small assortment of needles and sutures. I had been encouraged by seeing a slack-rope walker who put his feet in baskets, took a chair in one hand and an umbrella in the other, and walking to the center of the slack rope, placed the chair on the rope, sat down on the chair, opened and raised the umbrella, took a cigarette from his pocket, and lit it. I was confident after witnessing this feat, that I could train myself to do almost anything. I felt it would be far easier to train myself than hundreds of nurses whom I rarely saw.

I also hailed with joy the continuous Crossen sponge—a four-ply, five-yard long and six-inch wide strip of gauze, first introduced by Professor Crossen of St. Louis, Missouri. This long sponge was placed with one end fastened into a pocket of the sterile sheet covering the patient. By its use, it was impossible to leave a sponge in the abdomen, and it relieved the nurse from the worry of sponge-counting.

No one has appreciated hospital standardization, originated by Dr. Franklin Martin of the American College of Surgeons, more than I. Instead of taking to the hospital the entire operating room equipment prepared in my home, as I did for many years when I began to do surgery, I can now go to the humblest hospital and find perfect service.

A century ago the strongest argument against women in medicine was that its study would tend to make a woman coarse and barren of all feminine charms. No reasoning could be more fallacious, for the study of medicine develops tenderness, sympathy, tolerance, and benevolence. If it produces this effect in the case of the male physician, how much greater will be the result in that of the female. That the study of medicine in no way unsexes the woman doctor may be amusingly established by her attitude toward adoption.

The greatest mistake that I ever made was in the early years of my practice when I thought that my knowledge of sociology was sufficient for me to plan the placing of babies for adoption. It seems strange to me that I ever could have yielded to the temptation, but, when a childless woman fixed me with her baby-hungry eyes, I entirely forgot that I did not believe that mothers of illegitimate children ought to give away their babies. Although, occasionally, I might read in the newspaper something about baby farms or money traffic in babies, I did not understand how great a crime it was. To me, finding a welcome home for a baby was a delightful philanthrophy.

As my pen writes, I blush at some of my crazy escapades along this line. I never took Alice into my confidence when I went on a bye-baby-bunting hunt, although she knew that I had such aberrations. I was, therefore, surprised when one day, after a visit to the bank, she said, "I want you to get a baby for the teller down at the bank. He has a beautiful red-haired wife, and they are just crazy to adopt a baby. I have promised that you will get them one. I know that you can if you want to."

I promised to do my best, but I had nothing in sight at the time. After every visit to the bank, Alice came home telling how anxious the teller was for a baby, how he worried lest their home was too simple, and so on, until I dreamed of babies—babies on doorsteps, babies in baskets, babies everywhere.

It was during this unsuccessful baby-hunt that I was called to Muskegon to operate. I took a night train, arriving early in the morning. After the operations, while we were eating dinner, the late Dr. Lucy Eames remarked, "You don't know of anyone who wants to adopt a baby, do you?"

"Yes! Yes!"

I was all interest as she told about a brave little English lady who was so poor that she felt that an addition to her family would entail so many hardships for her other children that she had decided to give away her red-haired new-born baby if a good home could be found.

Here at last was the chance to please Alice, and to do the bank teller the favor of a lifetime. I immediately shifted my timetable and arranged to return on the afternoon train that would arrive in Chicago about one in the morning, instead of returning comfortably at night in the sleeper.

After the papers for releasing the baby had been signed, I started for the train, loaded down with the baby, a bag of diapers and milk bottles, and in addition, my own bag full of heavy instruments. The sleeper in which I had expected to return went through to Chicago without change of cars, but the afternoon train necessitated changing cars at Grand Rapids. The trip as far as Grand Rapids was promisingly uneventful, and the change of cars, though difficult, was accomplished. After that there was nothing but trouble. The baby became so noisy and unmanageable that even after it had had the four bottles of milk it was still screaming demoniacally.

I had telegraphed my cousin Clara to meet me at Englewood. When she saw me with the bag of wet diapers and jingling empty milk bottles, the baby, and my own huge heavy bag, she exclaimed, "Pete's sake! What have you brought?"

I put on a sickly grin and whispered, "The teller's baby."

She insisted that they would not like it if I came so late at night with the baby, but I thought it would be cute—the way babies have of coming at unexpected times. My heart was light even though my load was heavy as I climbed three flights of stairs to the teller's apartment. The prospect of getting rid of the baby made me cheerful, but the prospective parents did not share my feelings. They objected to having the baby left! I did not argue with them, for I thought if they spent the night with it, that by morning no one would be able to take it from them. So sure was I, that I blandly promised to come and get the baby whenever they wanted me to, if they should decide they did not want to keep it. They telephoned very early in the morning. When I took the baby away no one of us spoke. If they were more angry than I was, nothing short of a duel could have settled our differences.

I put the baby in the hospital and communicated with each of two women who had been importuning me to get her a baby. One wanted to wait another year to see if she might not conceive. The other, who had adopted a baby two years before, thought she had better not take a second one this year.

By this time I had lost every vestige of good sense. I remembered the repeated pleadings of a deaf and dumb couple who had thought that life would be perfect, in spite of their handicaps, if they had a baby. These people were not patients of mine, but they had a go-between, a wonderful woman, an ordained minister of a church for the deaf and dumb. She was one of four sisters whose parents were deaf and dumb. I had brought all four of these beautiful, college-educated women into the world, and had great confidence in their judgment. I gave the mutes the baby, and when I witnessed the joy of these foster parents I was repaid a hundredfold for the agonizing trip from Muskegon and the rebuff from people who had pestered me for months. I sincerely felt that I was a divine instrument answering the prayer of these people.

As long as the baby was little and in the home with its foster mother, everything was perfect. The parents took turns, during the baby's first year, in sitting up all night, watching the precious child lest it waken and call them. Strangely enough, the child became difficult to manage as soon as she was able to attend school. Her unseemly conduct soon became the talk of the neighborhood. The go-between reported to me this unbelievable state of affairs, and we resorted to all sorts of measures to reinstate discipline and order into the home. When things got shockingly bad, we turned the child over to the department of child welfare, and in a few weeks they located the child's own parents, who were now in comfortable circumstances and delighted to welcome their young daughter back home into the family circle with her own many brothers and sisters.

This desire to place babies for adoption is, I believe, a weakness quite common to women physicians, and from their confidences I find that they too, when the baby fever is on, act ridiculously. One very dignified woman physician related her experience in depositing a six-months, illegitimate baby on the doorstep of its own mother, who had married shortly after the baby's birth. An evening party had been prearranged, during which the mother, with feigned surprise, was to find the baby in a basket and feel so sorry for it that she would adopt the child. It was in late spring and did not get dark until nearly ten o'clock. Forgetting the long days, the doctor and her secretary started with the baby so early that they had to drive for nearly two hours before it was dark enough to leave the basket. The darkness, though necessary to conceal the identity of the bearer of the baby, made it difficult for the doctor to find her way across the unfamiliar back yard, and was the cause of her tripping on a barbed wire and landing on her face. The baby got such a jolt that its feet pushed through the end of the basket. Starting out again, the doctor stumbled on a step, but was able to land the baby at the door. Then, running on all fours like a frightened coyote, she reached her automobile, breathless from exertion and fear. Her secretary asked, "Why do you do such things, Doctor?"

The only answer was, "Because I'm such a stupid fool, but don't tell anybody."

Of all absurd make-believes, there is none more idiotic than that of a childless woman feigning pregnancy. Sometimes even a husband is tricked into the belief that he is the father of the baby of which his wife pretends to have been delivered. One of my cleverest patients, but withal a gloriously beautiful character, brought four babies, one every two years, into the home as her own, and her husband believed that he was the fortunate father of them all. After the children became adolescent their foster mother told them that they were adopted and that the father did not know it. It is almost unbelievable, but true, that they bore such love for their adopted mother that they joined her in keeping the truth from her husband, who died in happy ignorance of his inability to procreate.

Not taking the prospective father into the secret of a feigned pregnancy proved, on one occasion, to be a boomerang for one woman doctor. This friend of mine was distressed when she told me of a patient who had contracted syphilis and gonnorhoea from her unfaithful husband. In addition to his infidelity the husband had other sins quite as unforgivable. Hoping to hold him, the lady was so determined to have a baby that the doctor brought her one and supposedly confined her in her sumptuous home. When her husband was informed that he was a father, he told his wife that she could put nothing over on him, and that if it cost him a thousand dollars, he was going to call the most distinguished obstetrician he could find to examine her. The doctor told me of the woman's dilemma. I flew to her rescue with a program which now seems a dream to me rather than something I enacted as the star performer.

Four hours before the spy specialist arrived I prepared the patient for examination by cutting the skin on the patient's perineum and inserting three stiff silkworm sutures. Next, after I had injected both of her breasts with a solution of salt and water, these organs became so distended and sensitive that it was impossible to touch them. The lower abdomen was treated in the same way with the salt solution, until it felt as if she had been recently delivered. To complete the post-partum picture I introduced into the urinary bladder, urine obtained from a hospital patient delivered the previous day. A positive reaction in an Ascheim Zondek test establishes pregnancy beyond question; and the urine of a freshly delivered patient would yield this result.

The great consultant arrived and looked at, but would not touch the perineum, bristling with wiry sutures; he gently touched the tender engorged breasts, noted the thick body in the lower abdomen, and concluded by catheterizing the patient. The big bill that the suspicious husband paid did not distress him, I am sure, as much as the contemptuous look that the consultant of his own choice gave him. Although the integrity of this home was happily and perfectly restored, I am ashamed of my part in the hoax, but I had so often seen a young woman pay the price of bearing a bastard, the result of an indiscretion that meant nothing to the man, or of forfeiting her chances for motherhood because of a venereal infection contracted from her unfaithful husband, that I had longed to adjust her wrongs. I saw an opportunity and took it.

Often I am ashamed of my impulsiveness. Just a short time ago I exhibited a shocking lack of self-restraint. I love a movie and especially enjoy going with Alice, for we both prefer seats in the front where the view will be unobstructed. On this occasion we had just been seated when two women took seats immediately in front of us. The lady in front of me wore a hat that reared fantastically above her head and completely obstructed my view. When she made no move toward removing it, I leaned forward and whispered, "Kindly remove your hat. It interferes with my seeing the picture."

She switched her head and muttered, "I will not."

This hat had been built up as a component part of the lady herself, and removing it was like circumcising the wearer's head. Nevertheless, I lifted the hat. Grabbing her precious gewgaw, she rushed from the theater.

I remarked to Alice, "What a simple way to solve the hat-nuisance!" But five minutes later the usher came to us and asked Alice if she had removed a lady's hat.

"Certainly not!"

Then he asked me.

"Well," I said, "I asked the lady in front of me to remove her hat, and in leaning forward I might have touched it."

He looked amused, but said reproachfully, "You should have sent for me."

"If she returns, I will."

That incident will never be repeated.

Nothing excites the pride or stirs the emotions of a young medic more than being asked to make a sick call for a busy well-established colleague. Dr. Hickey Carr, who had indorsed my application for licensure, was the first physician to so honor me. During a few weeks' absence from Chicago she left in my care one of her obstetric patients who, near term, was waiting delivery in the hospital. This patient looked upon me as an interloper. Every day I suffered from her scorn and disapprobation. I sincerely hoped Dr. Carr would return in time to deliver her. One day to increase my confusion, she remarked, "You know so much, perhaps you could tell me when my labor pains will begin."

To meet her sally, I promptly prophesied. "Tomorrow morning at three o'clock."

Startled at my unhesitating reply, she continued, "Perhaps then, you can tell me when my baby will be born."

After an impressive silence I foretold the birth: "At ten o'clock, seven hours after you have been in labor," and to avoid further questioning, I left.

More to my surprise than to hers, her pains began exactly at the prophetic hour, and the baby was born at ten o'clock, fulfilling the horoscope. Although I insisted that my answers were only defensive jokes, this ridiculous incident changed my patient's attitude from contempt to veneration, and even before Dr. Carr's return, she insisted that henceforth I was to be her medical adviser. Nor could she understand the medical-ethics angle, even after I assured her that Dr. Carr's respect and friendship meant more to me than that of a hundred patients.

On another occasion in the absence of Dr. Carr I was guilty of taking most unethical revenge on one of her patients.

While a blizzard raged, and all means of transportation were fast failing, my telephone rang. A patient of Dr. Carr wanted me to come and see her at once.

Regarding all of her patients as important, I prepared to go. Poor, patient Kit was harnessed to the buggy, and with her head lowered to face the driving gusts of snow, her legs straining to drag the wheels through the drifts, we reached the home of the sick lady, where I was obliged to leave the horse across the street, since there was no hitching post in front of her house. I blanketed her, seized the carriage robes and my bag, and waded up to my knees in the sticky snow. The patient was sitting before a blazing grate fire in a becoming house gown, her slippered feet on the fender.

I am sure she detected no irony in my voice as I apologized, "I hope you suffered no discomfort while waiting for me. What can I do for you?"

She replied, "All day I have had kind of a ungh, ungh." (She imitated a hacking cough.)

I must have lost my self-control when I crossed the street, or it may have flown up the chimney with the sparks from the burning wood; at any rate it had utterly disappeared. I was glad not to have to reckon with it. "Well, well, we will see to that naughty cough!" I glowered ominously. "Take off all your clothes, and hop into bed."

She seemed alarmed. "Is it bad?"

I delayed answering. "We will see."

I made as thorough an examination as possible. I peered into her throat, turned back the upper eyelid, pulled her ears backward and forward, and gazed into them. I pinched, patted, and percussed every inch of her body; I drummed a tattoo on her chest and abdomen; I made a digital exploration of her rectum and vagina. When I could think of nothing more to do, I prognosticated, "You will feel worse tomorrow, but don't worry; these powders will fix you!" Thereupon, I gave her several superdoses of calomel to be followed with epsom salts, and I instructed her to stay in bed for two days.

As I unblanketed Kit and tramped about in the snow, I had no more resentment; I was even with the world. When I frisked into the house, Alice remarked, "That patient must have been pretty bad to have a doctor come out in this weather."

I explained, "She had nothing to do today so she sent for the doctor, but tomorrow she will be busy."

Several months later, one beautiful day in spring, Dr. Carr and I were having a little chat when she interjected, "By the way, I have always intended to ask you what you gave my patient last winter. She said it was wonderful for you to come in such a blizzard, and give her such a complete examination. She insisted she wasn't really sick when you came, but the next day she thought she was going to die. At any rate, you prevented her from having any real illness. What was it you gave her?"

I looked mystified and did not answer.

"Oh, you don't remember. It is of no importance. Never mind."

Dr. Carr never referred to the subject again, and I tried to forget that I, the doctor, had ever so completely disregarded my Hippocratic oath. More than that I was ashamed to have avenged myself on one of Dr. Carr's patients, for I was under deep obligation to her for befriending me in my early days in Chicago. Then too, I felt myself a part of Dr. Carr's family for I had delivered her when her beautiful daughter, now Mrs. Stephen Vincent Benèt, was born. Dr. Carr had lost two children before Rosemary's birth and I felt such responsibility for the health of this only daughter that I never went to the farm in the summer without taking her. "Aunt Alice" and Rosemary were both book-minded and very congenial. Remembering the great care that Dr. Carr exercised over Rosemary's diet I have laughed many times at Rosemary's answer when Alice asked, "What do you think your mother would say if she knew you were eating your thirteenth biscuit?"

With her mouth dripping with honey, she rolled up her big blue eyes and murmured, "Much I care."

In one respect Dr. Carr was unlike any other physician I have ever known: she never had a regular office either away from or inside her home. She explained this eccentricity by saying that patients did not like doctors' offices, furnished conspicuously with examining tables, instruments and bottles. She saw patients as guests in her home, used her bed for an examining table, and kept her medicines and instruments in a closet or in her doctor's bag. As she devoted her life to her patients, so did she throw open her home to them. She practiced medicine in a truly feminine way—in the home.

I can understand her attitude in this matter because I did much of my early operating in the home, and really enjoyed improvising and creating an operating room out of a stuffy parlor.

Many obstetricians try to make the public believe that twilight sleep cannot be given successfully in the home, but I know women physicians who have won laurels along that line.

In 1914, when I was devoting night and day to developing a routine method for administering scopolamine to produce painless childbirth, women physicians were eager to become my students.

One morning, Dr. Elizabeth Miner of Macomb, Illinois, appeared at the Women and Children's Hospital. She said that she had come to learn something about twilight sleep, and would remain with us until she was satisfied as to its safety and effectiveness. While we were talking, a patient passed through the iron gate of the fenced-in hospital grounds. She was shrieking like a Comanche Indian on the warpath. She yelled when she had a pain and did not stop between pains. We followed her to the preparation room where she was given at once an injection to produce twilight sleep. In ten minutes she was quiet and docile. In a half hour she was ready for the delivery table, smiling and obedient to every direction. The baby was born about an hour after the first dose of scopolamine had been given and, although free from pain, the mother was perfectly aware of everything that was going on. I explained to Dr. Miner that this was scopolamine analgesia and that another dose would have been required to produce anesthesia. Dr. Miner stayed to see many deliveries, but it was this first case that captivated her. She said that she would have been willing to spend many weeks and travel many miles to see that one case. To her it was a twentieth century miracle. She returned to her home town and used her knowledge of twilight sleep for the benefit of all the obstetrical patients in her very large country practice.

The contention that twilight sleep cannot be given in the home was emphatically disproved by our hard-working, as well as hard-headed and soft-hearted women physicians, Dr. Elizabeth Miner and Dr. Vesper Shaffer. Their hundreds of cases have proved conclusively that twilight sleep can be given in the home with even greater success than in the hospital.

Dr. Vesper Shaffer had a very large general practice of which the major part was obstetrics. She employed a full-time nurse to assist her in watching home deliveries and administering the hypodermic injections of twilight sleep.

Dr. Shaffer was a typical family doctor. When the man in one of her families had to have his enlarged prostate gland removed, he wanted to have the same surgeon that had operated on his wife's fibroid tumor, and Dr. Shaffer brought him to me.

One day a male surgeon solicited Dr. Shaffer for some of her surgery. He said, "I know you have Dr. Van Hoosen for your female patients, but how about sending me your male patients? Dr. Van Hoosen does not do prostatectomies."

"Oh yes, she does!" Then she added with emphasis, "What's more, the patient is able to urinate after the operation!"

Dr. Gertrude Thompson, who was present and overheard the remark, was greatly embarrassed and irritated. "Why did you have to say that?" she snapped.

"Well," Dr. Shaffer replied, unabashed, "it's true, and he asked for it!"

All of her patients regarded her as an important part of the family and were especially grateful to her for the long hours she spent in administering twilight sleep in the home.

The love and loyalty that the whole community in which she lived bore for her was shown in a dramatic way at her funeral.

She died fairly young of diabetes. Every seat in the little church on the northwest side of Chicago was occupied. All committee and overflow rooms in the basement were full; the windows were blocked with faces peering into the church; and every foot of ground within hearing distance was crowded by men, women and children. Three clergymen officiated: her pastor when she first came to Chicago, the brother of the nurse who lived with her and assisted in the deliveries under twilight sleep, and the presiding minister who, when his turn came to speak, gave a most unusual talk.

He began with, "Oh, I don't see how I can ever get along without her, and I know all of you feel as I do—I wish I had taken her more flowers—raise your hands, you who have been her patients."

The church was a sea of waving hands.

"Yes, those are the flowers, the loving service that she gave freely to all of us—I was just like you, for when I got into trouble, I always went straight to her, and left happy and smiling. What am I to do now?"

The ushers signaled for those who wished to say good-by to come forward and leave by the side door. Not one in all that congregation missed that last opportunity. Mothers passed, pressing their babies to breasts that heaved and shook with uncontrollable grief; old men knelt; strong men lifted little children that they, too, might see the face of the beloved. For many years Dr. Shaffer had given much of herself and taken little for herself, except the happiness of abiding in a thousand women's hearts and the joy of lifting the centuries-old fear of childbirth.

THE LAUGHING PATIENT

WHILE IN PEKING *I accompanied Dr. Emma Martin on a professional call on a young bride. We were ushered in and seated by the amah, a woman servant. Dr. Martin, in Chinese of course, asked her to expose her chest that she might listen to her lungs. To do so, the patient unfastened one silken embroidered jacket after another until she reached the bare skin. Throughout the call, the patient laughed constantly.*

I asked Dr. Martin, "What was the matter with the patient?"

She answered, "A vaginal discharge."

Puzzled, I queried, "Why did you make no other examination than that of the chest?"

"Oh," Dr. Martin explained, "this is the first time she ever saw a foreigner or a woman doctor. I felt I had done enough for one time. She will talk about this visit for the next three days and tell all her friends how funny we were."

"What!" I gasped. "Am I funny?"

"Why, yes," Dr. Martin said, "you are very funny. Didn't you notice that she laughed all the time?"

"But," I persisted, "in what way am I funny?"

"Well," she said, "first, there is your hair. It looks as if rats had nested in it. Then there are your shameless breasts, sticking out on your chest, instead of being bandaged close to the body. And worst of all, your feet. They look like gunboats."

I listened and began to understand why the Chinese children always followed us and laughed at every move we made.

19

CHINA VIA THE CORAL SEA

IN THE SUMMER of 1922, the year following Mother's death, I began to lay plans to take a trip to New Zealand, Australia, and the Orient because I had been advised to spend three winters in a warm climate to relieve my bronchial asthma, an unrecognized symptom of gall bladder disease. An interim between studying agriculture and taking up farming would enable Sarah to go; and I thought that Alice should have some trenchant pleasure as she was expecting to accompany Sarah to the farm and leave Chicago, which she loved so much that she had often said, "When I die, I want my ashes broadcast over the Loop."

My gall bladder ruptured in July, and an operation upset our plans for a time, but not for long. I was able to practice again one month after the operation.

In October we sailed from San Francisco on second-class tickets to Honolulu. On the boat to Honolulu we made friends with the owner of a bird store who had just made a buying trip to South America. She was returning with a large collection of parrots. As we were nearing port, quite unexpectedly a friend of hers came aboard our ship from the pilot boat. She introduced us to him and in about ten minutes he had found out that we were going to stay a month in Honolulu; and we had found that he had a furnished bungalow for rent, that the bungalow was opposite his home and very near the Moanna Hotel, fifteen minutes' ride to the city center by street car. The rental of the bungalow, by the month, was $50. We took it, sight unseen, and rode, bag and baggage, with him straight to our new home.

The bungalow was better than his description, for he had not told us of the papaya trees and the banana stalks in the back yard, or of the sweet-voiced Chinaman who passed our door every morning calling, "Flaws!," his arms strung with baskets of blooms so beautiful and so cheap that we wanted to buy all of them.

There were no mosquitoes or flies in Honolulu, and it was never too cold or too hot. Every day there was a sprinkle of rain from a passing cloud, that was accepted by us as a blessed baptism into this land of beauty and bliss. We cooked most of our meals because there were five of us to do it, and it was such fun to buy fruit we had never tasted, fish we had never before seen, and strange cakes of Chinese, Japanese, Filipino or Hawaiian make. Even to ride on the streetcar was a joy, for if every seat was full as the car approached, there were always seats for ladies, regardless of nationality.

Every time a boat entered or left the harbor, we missed much if we were not there to meet it or see it depart. We enjoyed the leis—sometimes a dozen around the neck of the departing passenger. Men and women, their arms hidden in blossoms, stood on the dock to sell these floral necklaces. Small black-skinned boys were climbing about, waiting for a chance to dive for the money that the passengers threw from the decks into the water. Over, above, and through it all was the music of the Hawaiian band, bidding godspeed to every departing guest, with the pleading strains of "Aloha Oe."

It was in the Hawaiian Islands that I first made a fearsome trip on a surf board. Here I first met a Filipino woman in her gauzy national dress. Here I first saw pineapples growing. Here I observed leprosy, and visited a leper colony. It was not the famous colony at Molokai, one of the Hawaiian Islands where all the inhabitants are lepers under the care of specialists, but the one just out of Honolulu. Here the majority of the patients were so nearly recovered that the physicians deemed them safe for parole. Many did some kind of labor in Honolulu or on the surrounding farms, at the same time continuing their treatments at the clinic.

At this parole clinic I sat by the side of the doctor while he treated more than three hundred patients during a short afternoon period. On the table in the clinic room were many trays of sterile needles, cotton, and skin disinfectants. Skilled technicians filled syringes with the prescribed doses of chaulmoogra oil and handed them to the doctor. An attendant called the patients by number. The women lifted their many voluminous petticoats and presented their buttocks for the deep intramuscular injections. The men, when their turn came, dropped their trousers. With this perfectly developed technique these hundreds of patients were treated in a minimum of time.

Here in the Islands I first beheld a volcano, approaching it through a forest of tree ferns. Here I first ate papaya, breadfruit, mangoes, and custard apples. Here I discovered hedges of the night-blooming cereus, and gazed in awe at a wonderful fire tree with its flaming red blossoms. One day we even came upon a row of African tulip trees in full bloom.

Not only in nature did we find such wonders, but in social relations as well—as if, out here in the Pacific Ocean, the millennium had arrived. A beautiful, tall young woman who was employed in the Board of Health, said to me with rising pride, "I am part Hawaiian; I have Hawaiian blood in my veins." At another time, a brilliant young man proudly claimed, "I am half Hawaiian and half Chinese." Tolerance, pride in achievement, appreciation of beauty, love of service to others, seemed to create about the people of the islands the atmosphere which nature herself seems to seek for growing and thriving.

The most delightful phase of the medical profession is to find that no matter how far the physician travels from his base, patients will be waiting for him. The first call I made in Honolulu was at the post office, where I was accosted by a former patient with, "The Lord has sent you! They say my appendix must come out, and here you are." The next week I performed a buttonhole appendectomy on her, and made delightful friends at the Queen's Hospital. Incidentally, I earned enough money to pay my passage to China.

Through this patient who was doing social service work, I was invited to give a lecture and demonstration clinic for the Honolulu welfare committee, which was just starting a prenatal clinic. I used the peel of a pamela, a fruit resembling a very large grapefruit, and a tangerine for models. Out of the pamela peel I cut a miniature pelvis, and on the tangerine I drew a face, and with those demonstrated the position of the foetal head in relation to the mother's pelvis, and the mechanism of labor. After the lecture, we measured the pelvis of some of the expectant mothers who were waiting in the clinic. I found that the Filipino pelves (with measurements six inches, external conjugate) were so small that we would expect the babies to be born alive only by Caesarean section. Yet, these tiny-pelvesed women had large families with no difficulty because the head of the baby was proportioned to the mother's pelvis. In the Chinese and Japanese, the pelvis is smaller than in American mothers (who have pelves eight inches, external conjugate); but the Hawaiian mother has a huge pelvis (nine or ten inches, external conjugate), and, as might be expected, an easy labor. Few of the Hawaiian women came to the clinics for prenatal instruction, for a large proportion of them still follow the tradition that it is the husband's duty to care for his wife in confinement. Hence, the Hawaiian bridegroom receives instruction in the delivery of the baby and the cutting of the cord.

After a five-weeks' stay we again embarked for China by way of the South Seas.

New Zealand, a land of dairying, presented a field of interest for Sarah, who made many side trips into the country to visit the farms and see the cattle. We planned to stay there only long enough for Sarah to study the farming.

Meanwhile, I made a visit to the hospital in Aukland to see

some of the surgery, and happened to find Dr. Kenneth MacKenzie operating. His technique was so good that when I was talking with him after the operating, I ventured, "I mean it as a compliment, and I hope you will understand me, for I must say that you operate more like a woman surgeon than any other man I have ever seen."

He replied, "Thank you for the compliment. I ought to operate like a woman, and am proud if I do, because I was taught by, and was assistant to a woman surgeon, Dr. Frances Ivans of Liverpool."

I had always been interested in that much-decorated woman physician who had done much commendable surgery during World War I, and it was almost like seeing her to meet one of her students.

We had great difficulty in getting passage from New Zealand across the Tasman Sea to Australia. On account of a strike, we had to sail third-class on a boat with a scab crew, or wait, perhaps for weeks, before we would have any other opportunity to sail.

Our third-class tickets put us in a cabin with eighteen berths including ours, all occupied. This cabin was next to the animal-like quarters, not even third-class, where they put some Chinese who came on board with twenty-one tickets handed in by one of the group. But when the boat was well on its way, the men were counted and there were twenty-three. This problem kept up an argument until we reached Sidney, where the twenty-three Chinese left the boat with the mystery unsolved.

It was a very rough passage, and Sarah and I, as usual, took to our berths. Despite the bad weather, the others went to the dining room and came back with tales of tablecloths dripping wet to prevent dishes from falling off the table, food inedible, and passengers intoxicated—altogether a wretched passage.

In Australia, where we spent three weeks, I was fortunate in meeting another very superior surgeon, Sir Alexander McCormack. I had heard so much about his skill that I went to his private hospital (he had just become emeritus at the large general hospital in Sydney) and saw him do a number of very difficult gall bladder operations with such care and thoroughness, as well as familiarity with pathological anatomy, that my admiration was excited. As an instructor and demonstrator he was profuse, and I envied the students who had been under his instruction.

He asked me to come the following Saturday to his clinic, but I wanted to see the Sidney Zoo, which covered an entire island across the harbor from Sydney, and was reached only by boat. Although we had visited all the zoos in Europe, we found this one far superior—really de luxe. The sea air, the walking, and the unfamiliar sights tired us, and we slept late the following (Sunday) morning. As I was finishing breakfast, our landlady came fluttering in, and announced with unfeigned surprise, "Sir Alexander McCormack is outside in his automobile to take you to his hospital."

I dressed quickly, and it was true—the great surgeon had come to take me on his morning hospital rounds. He introduced me to the patients, and gave me a short history of some twenty-five who were convalescing from their various operations. Then he instructed the chauffeur to take me for a ride while he went to the office to look over his mail.

The chauffeur, in his efforts to entertain, gave me such a delightful insight into Sir Alexander's character that when he again joined us, I felt that he was a colleague and not a stranger.

Instead of taking me back to my people, he announced that I was to go home with him for dinner. His home was on one of the highest points overlooking Sidney Harbor. Mrs. McCormack was away, but the grown son, with a friend, and the daughter were there. After a very good dinner, Sir Alexander said, "Who's going with Dr. Van Hoosen and me in the yacht?"

The son's friend was anxious to go, and walking down the steep hill, we found the yacht anchored in a little cove. After boarding, Sir Alexander took off his shoes and stockings, and himself steered the boat all over Sidney Harbor. It was the largest yacht on the harbor, and this, my first (and up to date, last) yacht ride was without a blemish. To make it truly exotic, when a little after 4:00 P. M. we were back in the cove, the butler had tea ready in the cabin—tea with delicious cakes and sandwiches, and gay Sir Alexander for company. The climax came when at my request I was escorted home in a sidecar!

We sailed from Sidney a month later by the Coral and South China Seas to Hong Kong on a Japanese boat, the *Yoshina Maru*. The boat was clean, and the meals beautifully served, with a different kind of fruit every day.

We traveled second-class, as usual, meeting fine people, some educated, some professional, and some wealthy. A sweet Australian young mother and her Japanese baby had a cabin near ours. After having married the Professor of Japanese in the University of Australia, from which she herself had a degree, the young woman was cast off by her parents. Hence the dishonored lady was on her way to Japan, to see whether her husband's parents would accept her and her baby, whose paternal chromosomes stamped him as Nipponese. The little lady took her meals in her cabin, devoting herself to her baby. I wanted to advise her to go to Honolulu, where all they expect of one is to belong to the human race, for which they have respect, regardless of color.

Like the Duke of Windsor, who once took this voyage from Australia to Hong Kong, we pronounced it a "dream voyage." We seemed to be drifting from one island to another, although we made few stops. At Thursday Island we saw pearl divers, and stores that were filled, room after room, with cabinets full of pearls. There were two stops in the Philippine Islands—one at Zamboango, and the other, Manila.

Arriving at Hong Kong, we made our first acquaintance with the Chinese, as one must pass through the Chinese quarter on the way to the English portion of the town. We stayed in a hotel until we could communicate with the mission in Canton, China, where we were planning to visit.

Bathtubs in foreign countries are often bizarre to Americans, but in Hong Kong we met with something entirely new. Visualize a porcelain jar about two and a half feet high, with a plug at the bottom. This jar, large enough for an adult to step in and squat, stood in the corner of the room, and invited the hotel guest to a bath. As I sat, embryo style, peering over the edge of that strange tub I laughed, for I had not yet learned that in just such a jardiniere the priests are placed in kneeling position for burial.

We did not dare to leave Hong Kong until we heard from Dr. Hackett, our hostess in Canton, especially as bandits were reported disturbing trains, and there was a war in that city. To our complete frustration, when we at last got a message to come by train, a second message came for us, "Better come by boat. Safer. Reports of bandits."

We went by train, however, and met no bandits. When we arrived at eight in the evening, Dr. Hackett and some of the missionaries were at the station to meet us. The trip to the mission necessitated traversing the diagonal of the city, first in rickshaws along the bund until we reached the old quarter of Canton, and then in sedan chairs to the mission. There were eight of us, making quite a procession. When we changed from the rickshaws to the sedan chairs, Dr. Hackett said, "Now the boys with the sedan chairs are from our own mission, and are perfectly reliable. You need not be afraid, no matter what happens. They will take good care of you, and my chair will be right behind yours."

We climbed into the chairs that were hoisted to the shoulders of the carriers, and started for the mission. The streets were so narrow that they did not seem like streets, but more like trenches or tunnels, with low Chinese homes or shops on either side. Carrying us was hard, grueling work, and I heard the carriers make strange, unearthly sounds, something between a grunt and a groan. The street paving was very uneven, and the carriers now and then stumbled, setting the chair in commotion. Periodically came a special grunting groan when the carriers shifted the chair from one shoulder to the other. Every now and then I discovered a hand touching the side curtains on the sedan chair, and a curious Chinese face peering into mine.

The days in Canton were full, for with lecturing to the students, operating at the medical school of which Dr. Hackett was founder and dean, going shopping and sightseeing, there was no time left. The exquisitely carved ivories, brocaded and embroidered silks were tempting, and we were told that we would not find such a variety in any other city.

From Canton we went to Shanghai, a short distance from which is Bethel, the large and busy mission conducted by Dr. Mary Stone, with whom we spent a few days. I had looked forward to seeing Dr. Mary Stone and Dr. Ida Kahn. At this time they were both at the peak of their careers. Their link with Michigan, my native state, and the University of Michigan, from which I had three degrees, had created between us a bond of love and interest.

These two Chinese women doctors, devoted to spreading Christianity, were pioneer medical women who owed their successful careers to their association with Miss Howe, who when a young girl living in Adrian, Michigan, had had a "call" to go to the heathen, and give her beautiful, comforting faith to them. She met with opposition, but undaunted, finally reached the Methodist mission in Kiukiang, China.

Shortly after Miss Howe began her missionary work, her Chinese teacher came to her in great distress. He told her of the ill luck of a family of Khans, descendants of Confucius, an exceptionally fine family. Mrs. Kahn had given birth to six girl babies, but since the family was influential he as go-between had arranged a desirable marriage for each one. The seventh baby proved also to be a girl. Fortunate as a go-between for the other six, he again succeeded in arranging a good marriage for the seventh. At the proper time the baby girl was arrayed in her red betrothal robe, placed in the red sedan chair, and carried across the fields to the home of the prospective bridegroom's parents. According to custom, just before the betrothal ceremony, her horoscope was read and—horror of horrors!—it indicated clearly that whoever plighted troth to this baby girl was cursed—his life subjected to grief and failure.

She was returned to her parents, not only unbetrothed, but unbetrothable. What would become of a girl without the possibility of future marriage? She would have to be sold as a slave, or made away with—unless—and this was the plan of the sensitive, kindly Chinese teacher, "Will you adopt her, Miss Howe? Will you save the baby's life? She is beautiful, and to you foreigners the horoscope makes no difference!"

When he brought the number-seven little girl, Miss Howe's heart was so touched that she adopted her. A number of years later, the missionary board made a rule that missionaries could not adopt children; however, it came too late to prevent Miss Howe's adopting several Chinese babies.

Ida Kahn, the number-seven girl baby, was soon ready for more extended education than she could receive in the mission school. Since she could not marry, but could be of much service to the Chinese as a physician, Miss Howe thought she should go to America to study medicine. Pastor Stone, a Chinese Christian minister of Kiukiang, had a little daughter, Mary, about the age of Ida. When he begged that Mary might go with Ida to America to study medicine, Miss Howe consented, and with the two girls returned to Michigan, where Mary Stone and Ida Kahn were educated, and received the degree of M.D. from the University of Michigan.

After graduating, the girls went back to Kiukiang, and together took charge of the hospital that had been built and equipped in memory of his wife, by Dean Danforth of the Northwestern University Women's Medical School, Chicago. For several years they worked together until Dr. Kahn, with Miss Howe, left Kiukiang to take charge of medical and missionary work in Nanchang, a day's ride on the train south of Kiukiang, farther into the interior of China.

Dr. Mary Stone remained at the Danforth hospital for a time, but wishing to establish a religious center in a more populous city, she with one of the missionary nurses went to Shanghai. To carry out their plans they needed money, friends, and land, as well as courage and faith. With courage and faith in abundance they set themselves to their task, and when I visited Bethel I was filled with amazement at what Dr. Mary Stone and her helpers had accomplished.

They had raised money and secured a large tract of land, on which they built a great tabernacle for religious services and a group of hospital buildings. There were many other buildings, a group of school buildings, homes for nurses and midwives, dormitories and workshops, a little city in itself. To appreciate Bethel one must do more than see the fine buildings and equipment. One should stay for a long time or make repeated visits to see the results of coordinated efforts to save bodies and souls; to bring habits of health to a country unversed in sanitation; to develop character and ambition by pleasure and faith.

Before leaving the United States I had been invited by Dr. Chi Che Wang, one of the first Chinese women to obtain a Ph.D degree, to visit her relatives in Soochow. From Shanghai we made a side trip to that beautiful city, where Dr. Wang's sisters, who conducted a private school, took us to visit a one-hundred-room Chinese home.

The hundred rooms through which we were shown were in twenty-five one-story houses separated by courts filled with flowering plants and shrubs, statuary, fountains, and rock gardens.

A Chinese family is composed of the father, the mother, the unmarried children, the grandparents, and the married sons with their families. These groups have their own rooms and servants, each occupying one or more houses and courts. There is no common dining room or communal apartments. Contrary to what one might think, this close family housing, instead of inducing intimacy, tends to develop individuality.

The family that lived in this wonderful home was away, and Dr. Wang's sisters had to obtain permission for us to see it, as it belonged to one of the wealthiest men in Soochow. In all the United States there is no building that could give one an adequate idea of such a place. It seems strange that no one in our country has ever built a summer resort or an Oriental museum on such a scale, after such a model.

From Shanghai we sailed up the Yangtze River to Kiukiang, stopping for one day at Nanking. The boat left the dock at 11:00 P.M. and was well on its way when I was suddenly awakened by great screaming and yelling, so loud that it must have come from the throats of many people. I slipped on my kimono and sallied forth to see if after all our ocean travel, we were going to be drowned in the big dirty river. I met an officer on deck and inquired, "What in the world has happened?"

"Nothing," he said, "only some Chinese leaving by a small boat and others being taken on board."

The top deck of our boat was occupied by the foreign passengers and the lower, by the Chinese. I leaned over the rail and watched the excitement until the boat moved on and quiet again reigned. Many stops were made before we reached Nanking, but always there was the same furor and excitement while the Chinese were disembarking or boarding the ship.

Many think of the Chinese as a stolid people, but the little knowledge I gained while in China as to their temperament was that they were the most excitable and temperamental people I had ever met. One case particularly interested me. While in the mission at Kiukiang, I slept on the second floor, very near the high compound wall. One night after I had gone to bed, I heard a Chinese woman on the other side of the wall, yelling as loudly as a football fan. I could not understand her, and tired after a busy day of work and sightseeing, I fell asleep, but was wakened several times during the night, by this woman who was still yelling, with no abatement in force or frequency.

In the morning, at breakfast, the missionaries grumbled, "Wasn't that terrible last night? I am afraid you couldn't sleep."

I wanted information. "Who was it made such a fuss?"

One of them volunteered, "Oh, a woman whose baby died of smallpox."

After breakfast I met Dr. Tseo, in charge of the hospital, who in most sympathetic tones, told me how this woman, when over forty years of age, had had her first baby—how the two-year-old baby had contracted smallpox and died. Dr. Tseo said, "I just lay awake and suffered for the poor soul. She may never have another child, and this was a boy. I wanted to scream and mourn with her."

Dr. Tseo was from a very prominent family. Her father had held a political position of honor and possessed much wealth, as evidenced by his many concubines.

I had looked forward to this visit at Kiukiang with Dr. Tseo, who had been my first assistant at the Willard Hospital, Chicago, for one year. Before coming to assist me, she had attended the Northwestern University and the University of Michigan, had taken her medical degree from Rush Medical College in Chicago, served an internship in Bellevue Hospital in New York City, and a residency in the New England Hospital for Women and Children. No Chinese woman had ever come to America for a medical education and returned to China so well-equipped as this slender, high-bred Chinese girl.

While I was with her in Kiukiang, as she was anxious to do as much operating as possible, we operated nearly every day. On the last day, we operated on fifteen patients—taxing the capacity of the Danforth Hospital.

I was profoundly impressed that here in China the two men who had meant so much to me in my early professional life, Dr. William Quine and Dr. I. N. Danforth, had each built a hospital in memory of his wife—Dr. Danforth in Kiukiang, and Dr. Quine in Ching Kiang.

The romance in Dr. Quine's life gave me a glimpse into the idealism and the chastity of his character. While a student in Rush Medical College he became acquainted with Miss Lettie Mason who was also studying medicine but at the Woman's Medical College of Chicago. They would have married, but Miss Mason had signed up to become a missionary and would not break her word. She did, however, promise like Rachel of old, to return in seven years and marry him.

Less than a year in foreign fields found her, a victim of pulmonary tuberculosis, returning to America on board a steamship with a metal casket in case of her death en route.

Dr. Quine met and married her at San Francisco. By slow stages he took his bride, not able to leave her bed, back to Chicago. She grew daily worse. Her chest was filling up with pus, but her condition was such that no surgeon would operate.

It was then that her devoted husband steeled himself and, without an anesthetic, plunged a knife through her chest wall. The imprisoned pus gushed forth. The tide was turned. She recovered and for twenty-five years lived in sweet communion with her brave and loyal savior.

From Kiukiang we made a side trip to the mountain resort of Kuling, taking sedan chairs and spending an entire day on the journey, most of the time climbing the mountain. After crossing a long stretch of lowland before getting to the foot of the mountain, the bearers doubled, with four men in front and four at the back. They climbed carefully and steadily. Some of the paths seemed too narrow to be safe even for goats, but our bearers, with their straw-sandaled feet, never hesitated or slipped. Often the chair in which we were seated extended out over a chasm hundreds of feet deep, and I tried not to look down, lest any dizziness on my part upset the equilibrium of the bearers. The mountain side was gay with pink and yellow azaleas, and a close-up of those orchid-like masses of bloom was worth some risk.

We arrived safely and spent the night with a missionary. In the morning I wakened in a whirl of dizziness that lasted for a couple of hours, but disappeared when I was able once more to climb into the sedan chair. With closed eyes and resignation to the worst, we began the descent.

It seemed best to go from Kiukiang to Nanchang, as Nanchang was then more accessible than it would be at any other point in our trip through China. At Nanchang we had planned to visit Dr. Ida Kahn, who was waiting impatiently for us.

We left Kiukiang by train, early in the morning, and arrived in Nanchang around 6:00 P.M. Dr. Ida was at the train to meet us, not with cap and bells, but with sedan chairs and firecrackers. There were six sedan chairs, mine leading the procession, while walking behind us were boys with long poles wound with firecrackers.

After crossing the river we started to go through the town, and the firecrackers were set off. The streets at once became jammed with Chinese, young and old, to see the foreigners go by. When we reached the hospital compound under the arched entrance bearing the hospital sign, there stood Mother Howe, then a woman over sixty, with white, white hair. Clustered round her were the Chinese nurses in grey uniforms and white caps, collars and aprons. They looked like birds as they waited in that lovely setting for us to arrive.

Dr. Kahn had wonderful success in growing roses. The compound was like a nursery, for besides a large rose garden, tiny white roses covered the compound walls and the sides of some of the brick buildings.

When she took me through the hospital, I was impressed with its order and cleanliness, and especially, with a fine big sterilizing apparatus for water, utensils, and surgical materials.

A few days after this, they asked me to operate on a large tumor. After putting on my cap and gown, I entered the operating suite. The first thing that I noticed was a block of four steps about six feet wide and four feet high. These steps sparkled with row on row of large two-gallon brass teakettles filled with water—sterile cold, sterile warm, sterile hot—it was a beautiful sight. I looked around and saw the shining big sterilizer of American make, unused, and asked Dr. Kahn, "Doesn't the sterilizer like China?"

She explained, "It cannot be run without gas, and since we have none, we have never been able to use it. It serves only to remind us of what China must work for."

I begged that I might take home with me one of those gorgeous brass kettles, and now when I read the newspapers and sense what has happened to this beautiful medical religious center and others, including Dr. Mary Stone's beloved Bethel, I feel that the big brass kettle is not large enough to contain my tears for precious China.

There was a beautiful relation between Mother Howe and her adopted daughter, Ida. One day at the dinner table, Mother Howe started to tell us something, but was stopped imperiously by Dr. Ida. Again Mother Howe made an unsuccessful attempt, but Dr. Ida said, "Mother Howe, I know what you are trying to tell, and I will not allow it." Seeing Mother Howe's great disappointment, we begged Dr. Ida to relent, and after much coaxing, she consented.

Mother Howe, in the gayest of moods, told the story—"When Dr. Ida was practicing in Tientsin and doing some government work, the President of China, with great dignity and in accordance with the customs of such an occasion, came to Tientsin and offered her his hand in marriage—but Dr. Ida refused."

Mother Howe had lived to see the baby girl with a bad horoscope turn down the highest marriage offer that a Chinese woman could receive. Though Dr. Ida had discouraged Mother Howe's telling the tale, it was evident that she took satisfaction in having overridden at least one of the superstitions which thrive almost with the rice in China.

It was not in France but in China that I learned what an art cooking could become. It was in China that I made the acquaintance of "tea eggs," made by boiling eggs in strong tea and gently cracking the shells so that the taste permeates the whole egg. Then there were lime-baked eggs called "one hundred-year-old eggs," made by covering the eggs with a thick layer of lime. With this treatment they can be preserved for any length of time, and become almost like gelatin. The Chinese also introduced us to the custom of dropping tiny pigeon eggs into a bowl of boiling soup and eating them with the soup.

Dr. Frances Heath told me of an experience she had while making a call on a convalescent patient, wife of a government official. She came in just as refreshments were being served to several guests who were calling on the sick lady. Dr. Heath was enjoying the dainties that were being passed when she noticed a bowl of embryo birds. The ladies put the tiny birds into their mouths, and, with their tongues, skilfully extracted the legs and bills, swallowed the bodies, and spat out the bills and legs. Dr. Heath was versed in Chinese customs and manners, and she knew she must partake of these embryo birds. But—could she? Every moment, the bowl of birds was coming nearer. Closing her eyes, she put a bird into her mouth. She said, "I never knew a bird could have so many bills and legs, but finally they reduced themselves to the proper number, and I spat them out, opening my eyes, surprised that I was still alive!"

On one occasion we were fed with duck that had been boned, and when cooked, looked like any duck that had not been boned. It was cut in slices and served like bread or meat loaf.

Dr. Kim, who at one time gave lectures in the United States on domestic science problems, entertained Jane Addams and our party at her home in Peking. Among the refreshments she served were chicken sausages made of finely-cut chicken meat stuffed into small chicken cases. I have never tasted a greater delicacy.

I never acquired a taste for melon seeds, though the Chinese seem to love them. However, I tried more than once water chestnuts, bamboo sprouts, bean sprouts, and even watermelons with green rinds and centers of a rich yellow color.

In Shanghai we had water-buffalo butter. It was as white as lard, but of a very delicate taste. The milk of the water buffalo is one of the richest, containing eleven per cent fat. Not unlike the milk of our Holstein breed, it has very little coloring matter, yet the percentage of fat is three times that of the milk from the Guernseys.

On the way to Peking we stopped over a few days in Hankow, staying in a very comfortable Seventh Day Advent Mission filled with missionaries on furlough, businessmen, and tourists passing through like ourselves. It was here that I became acquainted with Mother Adams, who had come to China as a girl, under the Inland Mission, but who, after her marriage, became anxious to work under the Baptist Mission Board of the United States. Mother Adams, who had about a dozen children, finally secured appointment under the Baptist Board after many trips to the

United States. For many years she worked in their mission field, a short distance from Hankow, until her husband died.

Mother Adams had built a beautiful little fenced-in cemetery lot for him. His grave was built of cement, with a headstone commemorating his life and work. She was in hopes that the Chinese might imitate this style of burial instead of following the traditional sloppy hit-and-miss system of burying the dead in the spot where they had been born.

The most outstanding, surprising, and never-to-be forgotten sight in China is that of the graves, mounds of earth somewhat conical in shape, literally sprinkled over China—in cultivated fields, in the middle of public roads, in front and back yards, sometimes a number in a group, sometimes quite isolated. They are on the hillsides and in the swamps. There are no cemeteries in China; instead, China is one vast burial ground.

All of Mother Adams' children became missionaries, and after her husband's death she returned to the United States, where she accepted a position as housemother at one of the large eastern universities. The boys idolized her, but after a few years she was so fearful that she might die in the United States and that it would not be possible to be buried by the side of her husband in the carefully kept little cemetery that she returned to Hankow, China, where she gave advice and encouragement to the passing missionaries.

At last, Peking! The Methodist mission gave us a suite of rooms with a bath in the Sleeper Davis Hospital, and we took our meals in the compound. Looking out over the compound wall on that first day (and any day thereafter) we could see a large group of camels. From that time I loved Peking and my love increased day by day. Alice, who had never become sufficiently enamored of any country or city to care to stay long in it, said after two months' sojourn in Peking, "I think I could stay here—always."

I wish I could formulate the charm of Peking! It may be the camels that one sees loping in slow procession through the streets; or perhaps the moats filled with pink lotus blossoms surrounding the Forbidden City; or the wall surrounding the city, on the top of which one strolls in the soft summer evenings; or the Great Wall not far away, climbing interminably up and down, a great monument of the past, a curiosity of the present; or the summer palace, a fascinating exhibition of what the Chinese still contribute to the field of art.

Perhaps the charm lies in the theaters that have produced a Mei Lan Fang. Whatever it is, the charm is intangible but ever-present. One feels it sitting in the park watching the passers-by—young men, with their ankle-length, delicately tinted, high-necked silk coats; young women, with their gay trousers, and kimono-like upper garments; children, with their fancifully-cut hair and beautiful naked bodies; old men, with their long beards; old women, dressed in gay, red clothes; workers in blue full trousers, with bare backs and chests; women with bound feet; children with fancifully-made slippers; men with satin, soft-soled slippers; laborers with grass sandals; men with fans; women with umbrellas; men wearing pigtails; women with elaborate glossy puffs and decorative hairpins.

The missionaries spared no pains in giving us intimate glimpses into the daily lives of the Chinese. I was with Dr. Emma Martin, our missionary hostess, when she made a call on one of the concubines of the Little Emperor, and while waiting, was entertained with refreshments and Chinese music by his uncle.

During my visit to Peking the Peking Woman's Medical College effected a merger with the Shantung Christian College at Genanfu, and I was invited to give the address to the last graduating class of that now defunct school. Moving the college to Genanfu, almost a day's ride from Peking, and organizing classes as part of the curriculum of the Shantung Christian College, was a great responsibility, carried almost entirely by Dr. Frances Heath, Acting Dean of the Woman's Medical College, and Professor of Gynecology. She was also head of the Sleeper Davis Hospital in Peking. As I was to be in China another month, I offered to assume the surgical work in the hospital, and suggested that she go to the seashore and take a rest. This gave me the rare opportunity of teaching the Chinese interns surgery.

One of them, Dr. Knei Chen Shen, did her first Caesarean section during the month that I took over the surgery. A year later she came from China, and served an internship under me in the Frances Willard Hospital of Chicago.

My experience with Chinese women doctors has filled me with admiration for their character and their fine medical work. I know few Chinese men, and almost none well enough to be a judge of them; but I have trained many Chinese women, and though they have great individuality, I have never been disappointed in any one of them, for all have made good.

While I was in Peking, Dr. Heath was obliged to go to Shantung on business, and asked me to look after General Yin, who had heart and kidney disease, and might die during her absence. She instructed me to listen to his heart every day and to keep him comfortable.

She said the most worrisome duty she had to perform for the Chinese was to foretell the hour of a patient's death, for if the physician turned out to be a false prophet and the patient should die in bed, some very lowly person must be found to dress the corpse and place it in the casket. For this reason she impressed upon me the importance of recognizing the signs of death in time for General Yin, shrouded in his costly robe, to die in his coffin. Long before death the Chinese buy the burial robe and casket, an acceptable present to one approaching old age. Dr. Heath had even shown me the General's burial robe of yellow satin, heavily embroidered, with many beautiful pearls set into the design.

So it was with a feeling of towering responsibility that I assumed charge of General Yin. I went in a rickshaw with the amah as interpreter, and always found the General sitting on the kang with his first wife beside him and the cunning little concubines dancing attendance.

In order to examine the General's heart I had to climb upon the kang, a platform two and one-half feet high and six or eight feet square, heated in winter by fires lighted underneath. To sit gracefully or even comfortably on that flat surface calls for practice and perhaps heredity. Should I sit on my legs, folded beneath me, or stick them out straight in front? Before my training in kang-sitting was finished Dr. Heath returned, and I was happy to shift the responsibility of foretelling his death.

The General did die not long after the Doctor's return, after she had given the family notification so that, resplendent in his flaming yellow accouterments, he died in his coffin, made of wood so heavy and so thick that it took many men to lift it. The mouth of the rooster, kept for days in reserve, took the last breath from the mouth of the dying man, and at the funeral the rooster was strapped to the top of the coffin, to help the spirit of the General find its way back from the grave.

It is a very ancient custom among the Chinese not to allow the sick to die in their beds. Many, of course, may not be so rich or provident as General Yin and may not have ready and waiting a coffin, a burial robe, and the rooster. If no coffin is at hand, a water-bed is set up in the principal apartment of the home and as soon as the hour of death has been foretold by the soothsayer or the doctor, the dying patient is placed upon it.

This water-bed consists of three boards supported on trestles or benches and covered with a mat. As soon as the sick man has been laid on the water-bed, his wife or daughter-in-law wipes his body clean with lukewarm water, shaves his head and face, and puts on fresh clothing in order that he may enter the spirit world, clean and in neat attire. The moribund body is now covered with a sheet and left to breathe its last, quietly.

If the dying man has not been placed in his coffin before his death, the coffining is performed at a propitious time somewhat later, and with ceremonies almost as elaborate as those of the funeral, which takes place a month or more after death.

A week or two later the Doctor took me to call on the son of the dead General. As we approached the inner court, I heard weird sounds, the wailing of the concubines, upon whom was the onus of this perfunctory mourning during the thirty days before the funeral and burial. They wore the mourning vestments, long sack-like garments of unbleached muslin with raw edges, and bandages of the same material around their heads. We were led past the huge, closed coffin, in front of which was a small table loaded with the food for the dead—sweetmeats, nuts and little delicacies. Yet even though the casket was thick and heavy, and the corpse had been surrounded with sweet-scented herbs before it was closed, I could catch that unmistakable odor, the odor of dissolution.

The saying, "If you see one city, you have seen them all," is far from true in China, for each one has its own charm and characteristics. Tientsin, where I spent a short time with Dr. M. I. Ting, another University of Michigan graduate doing a big work in China, is not like Peking, Soochow or Canton. It is, perhaps, more like a small Shanghai.

Dr. Ting, and also Dr. Wang of Shanghai, always used a horse and closed carriage, when making calls or attending to business. While in Tientsin, I went with Dr. Ting to make a professional call, and to my surprise, when we arrived at the patient's home, the driver and the footman who always accompanied us, proceeded not only to take the horse out of the shafts, but to unharness and lead it about until we were ready to return. Then they harnessed the horse, put it back into the shafts, and we went on our way. At every street corner the footman descended and led the horse around the corner.

As fond as the Chinese seem to be of dogs, birds, chickens, horses and sheep, they seem to have little interest in cows. The Chinese do not drink cows' milk, but often the old and feeble, as well as the babies, nurse breast-milk, whenever possible. I learned that poor women went from door to door of the well-to-do, to allow some ailing person to nurse their breast milk. I have seen a mother, in the space of a half hour, nurse her two-month-old baby, her child of two, and another child of four years of age.

In some parts of China there is a disease known as osteomalacia, due to a deficiency of lime and characterized by a softening of the bones. When attacked, the patient actually becomes shorter in stature, and as the disease advances, the pelvic bones may collapse under the body weight, and the pelvic outlet becomes narrowed to the extent that birth through the natural passages is impossible.

I had studied the literature of such cases, but had never seen one. That I might have actual experience in observing this rare disease Dr. Martin planned to take me to Shensi, a province in the middle west of China.

Starting early in the morning, we traveled by train all day, arriving in the evening at a town south of Peking. Here we spent the night at an inn, and the next day journeyed again by train from eight in the morning until five in the evening. On leaving the train, Dr. Martin hired three rickshaws: one for our bags, and one each for ourselves. Our rickshaw boys had thirty miles to travel before reaching Taiku, our destination, where we were to stay over Sunday. They made the trip over none-too-good roads in five hours, at six miles an hour, never running, and stopping to rest only at tea shacks along the way.

Sunday morning after our arrival at Taiku, Dr. Hemingway, in charge of the mission hospital, had assembled many of these osteomalacic cases for me to see and examine. In addition, there were in the mission a boy in need of an operation for appendicitis, and a missionary who needed a gynecological operation, as well as an operation for painful bunions. We devoted the time from 5:00 to 10:00 A. M. Monday morning to this surgery, leaving as soon as the operating was finished.

After riding all the rest of the day in a bus, by evening we reached the next mission hospital. Here, traveling by Pekin cart, we saw more cases of osteomalacia in the homes of the patients. As the weather was fine, and I was not accustomed to sitting on my legs or with them extended, as is necessary in a Pekin cart, I sat in front, hanging my legs over the shaft.

Another day's bus ride brought us to Sianfu, capitol of Shensi, where, although there was a law against foot-binding, I do not remember seeing any women without bound feet.

On the return trip Dr. Martin and I parted company at the junction, a day's ride from Peking, since she wanted to take a little vacation at Kuling, while I, on a third-class ticket, traveled all day alone. I chose a seat in the extreme rear of the coach where I could see everything that happened to the passengers, who interested me more than those on any other trip I have ever taken. The majority did not use the seats to sit on, but sat on the tops of the backs, their feet on the seats. Many carried rolled-up mattresses which they deposited on the seats, or in the aisles, for people to stumble over. One man climbed up and took a nap on the baggage carrier, at the side of the coach, high above the seats. Another passenger, a woman, came in with her mattress, a baby and a large watermelon, and spreading the mattress on the floor under a couple of seats, lay down on the mattress. Holding her year-old baby in one arm, with her free hand she dug a hole in the watermelon, and during the entire trip she and the baby either slept, or ate handfuls of watermelon. There was a great deal of chattering, some smoking of water pipes, a laborious pastime, and considerable eating, as at every station there was an opportunity to buy delicacies.

Anticipating my thirst, Dr. Martin had taught me to say in Chinese, "cheeschway" (that is the way it sounded) meaning bottled water. The train boy had been through several times with brass kettles filled with hot tea water, or a hot, wet turkish towel on which the passengers in turn, wiped their hands and faces. As the day advanced, it grew warmer and warmer, and as I was beginning to get thirsty, I stopped the boy as he passed. "Cheeschway," I called. He bustled away and soon returned with my drink, but that one word had awakened the whole coach to a realization of my presence. I was at once bombarded with questions from every side, but I could only shake my head in deep regret that my vocabulary was limited to one word—"Cheeschway."

On my return to Peking I went to Tehchow in Shantung, to stay a few days with my old students, Dr. Emma Tucker, and her husband. There I met Dr. Lois Pendleton, a clever surgeon, who had a hospital full of interesting patients.

We did some extremely unusual and difficult operations. Dr. Tucker, who had been living in China many years, was keenly alive to what would interest foreigners. It was she who showed me how the women in the country, instead of dressing the newborn baby, put it unwashed in a sack containing several cups of sand. They tied the sack under the baby's arms and frequently changed the sand. This custom often resulted in infection of the navel, and death from tetanus.

We called on another Chinese woman living in the country, and as we were sitting on the kang, I felt our hostess' hand under my dress, running up my leg.

Dr. Tucker noticed it and told me, "Never mind, the woman is just curious as to what you're wearing under your dress! Many times I've stripped to the skin for a group of Chinese women to show just what kind of underclothing I wore."

We passed a small house where a woman was standing on the roof, screaming at the top of her voice. I said, "Dr. Tucker, what does that mean?"

"Oh," she answered, "that woman is displeased with the way her husband treats her, and she is telling it to the world! She will stand there on that roof all day long, until by night she will be so hoarse that she cannot make a loud noise."

I looked at the woman and exclaimed, "Whoever thought the Chinese were a stolid, unemotional people?"

Back in Peking, this great Oriental city, all our days were happy, except the month that Alice was dangerously ill with an intestinal infection. We had been strict during our stay in China not to eat any uncooked food, or drink unboiled water. The missionary homes where we had stayed had made it easy for us, but in Peking, we found a place serving delicious ice cream that I erroneously thought had been cooked before freezing, rendering it harmless. When I suddenly realized that eating ice cream might be the easiest way to get an infection, it was too late.

For several weeks Alice was too ill for us to be certain as to the outcome, and my poor Sarah prayed that her mother might be spared us for at least ten more years. Dr. Heath was a most skillful surgeon, but her ability in internal medicine was especially outstanding, and if not for her, I am sure Alice would never have lived through that terrible attack.

Then too, Alice's rickshaw boy, Mah, must have stimulated her by his devotion. When we began sightseeing in Peking, Dr. Martin advised us, "Each one of you pick out a hospital rickshaw boy, and keep the same boy while you stay."

I selected a big fellow with a pock-marked face, but Alice selected a man in his early twenties, a beautiful Atlantean runner. Alice's boy, Mah, had been a daily delight to her as he picked up the rickshaw shafts and trotted off with the lightness and grace of a professional athlete.

When Alice was taken sick, she said, "Now I want you girls to let Mah take you every now and then so that he will not miss out on account of my sickness." Before we had had a chance to ride with Mah, he sent Alice a lovely water hyacinth. We were deeply impressed, and each made an effort to take Mah, and increase his tip. But it mattered little; Mah continued to send Alice daily floral offerings.

In despair she entreated Dr. Martin, "Please tell Mah not to spend his money that way."

But Dr. Martin laughed, "Why, you are old; too much cannot be done for old people in China, and Mah is very happy so to honor you. Don't make him miserable."

So this delightful custom of honoring the old went on, and we lagged after, with vain efforts to keep up with extra tips and extra trips until the day came when Dr. Heath thought that Alice could travel again. We were to go by train to Tientsin, and from there by boat to Kobe, Japan. Alice had the hospital Ford take her to the station, where Mah met her, lifted her out of the Ford into the rickshaw, and with every muscle in perfect harmonious action, sped lightly through the station. He saw her safely into the car, and to the reserved seat that had been covered by Mah before our arrival with a blanket of tuberoses. Alice turned to find him, but he had disappeared, never to be seen again.

THE PHANTOM SIX

WHILE DEVELOPING *twilight sleep for use in obstetrics, I spent the greater part of almost every night in the Women and Children's Hospital, ten miles from my home. When, in the wee small hours, I stepped into my Kimball electric car, I often worried lest I might fall asleep. With my horse and buggy no harm would have resulted, but even a slow-moving electric demanded alert reflexes. One night I left the hospital at 2 a.m. but was keeping close watch of myself fearful that I might fall asleep at the steering bar.*

Suddenly, at 45th and Michigan Avenues, there appeared directly in front of me a huge grey elephant. I stopped the car, for I was certain that I must be alseep. I clapped my hands, pounded my legs and pinched myself, but elephants continued to pass, one after another, each one smaller than the last, until the sixth and final one was just baby size.

Now thoroughly awake, but believing that I had napped and dreamt of elephants, I hurried home and went directly to bed.

The next morning Alice awakened me by calling, "Come to the window—look!"

There, passing the house, were my elephants of the night before, part of a small circus in the neighborhood.

20

JAPAN: CAUGHT IN THE 1923 EARTHQUAKE

WHEN WE BOARDED the boat at Tientsin to go to Kobe, we had little realization that we would never again be able to see the same beautiful China. And if we could have realized that Japan would so ruthlessly destroy China, as she has in these less than twenty years since that time, I fear we would never have taken even a peep into Nippon.

The passage from Tientsin to Kobe, like that from Australia to China, was a halcyon, Oriental-flavored voyage.

We had planned to go to Kyoto and Nara for a few days, and then on to Yokohama; from there, up to Nikko, where we would remain two weeks, and then back to Yokohama to board the Empress of Asia, sailing for Vancouver. On leaving Kyoto for Yokohama, as I got into my berth I said to my family, "I do not want to see any more ivory or jade or any more pagodas or temples. I would like to see the Japanese people as they really live." Little did I realize that on the following day I was to get my wish!

We arrived in Yokohama about seven o'clock the next morning. We were up and dressed early enough to enjoy passing through groves of feathery bamboo, past dashing streams of water and small lakes pink and thickly growing lotus blossoms. Green grass, cultivated fields and the absence of conical shaped graves made us realize we were not in China, even though we saw a pagoda occasionally, or a temple. On arriving at the station, an American Express boy took charge of our baggage, and we went directly to the Grand Hotel. There we enjoyed an American breakfast with cereal, griddle cakes and ham and eggs.

The train we were taking to Tokyo left at eleven o'clock. I wanted to leave the hotel at ten, but the American Express agent said not to worry; it would not take more than fifteen minutes to go to the station. I became increasingly anxious to leave.

My sister said, "What's the matter with you? You always tell us when we are on vacation that it doesn't matter if we miss a train or two."

"Not this time," I protested, and worried the American Express agent until he finally sent for the taxi. When we were about to leave, he came running out with a handful of letters, twenty-three in all, and gave them to me, one at a time, reading each address as he did so. I may have kept a calm exterior, but I was boiling inside with impatience. At long last we were sitting in the station with fifteen minutes to wait before the train would pull out.

The ride to Tokyo took less than an hour, and we arrived three minutes before noon. We were following the American Express boy who took our bags down into the station hotel lobby, when suddenly I heard the noise of noises. It came from above and from below; it closed in on all sides. The elevator near which I was standing shook its chains like an enraged gorilla. My feet felt queer.

Sarah seized my arm and cried, "Earthquake! Hurry!"

We grasped each other by the arm and plunged towards the open door, twenty feet away. Like a string of children playing crack-the-whip, we swayed this way and that, now touching the floor, now rising as though on the crest of a wave. Breathless and groaning, we at last reached the open door just in time to see a six-story stone building across the street collapse like a house of cards, and a cream-colored brick building next to it split open in many places from top to bottom, while the window glass showered down upon the pavement. We made one more struggle through the door, and as suddenly as the quake had come, it was over.

All was quiet. Alice was outwardly hysterical, and the rest of us, inwardly. We clung to each other, uttering unintelligible words. When we finally regained an outward calm, another earthquake began. I saw the Japanese people all about us squatting, and I followed suit, ordering the others to squat. Alice refused, and when the quake was over, she said, "If I had squatted, I would never have been able to rise again."

A plot of green grass with trees, in the center of the plaza in front of the hotel, afforded a place of safety for us and many others. This first earthquake had been of the vertical type, lasting four minutes. Others of the horizontal type and of seconds' duration followed. I timed them, as we do labor pains, on my watch, now every two minutes, now every five minutes, now with an eight-minute interval. In the two days following the first quake, I was told that seven hundred quakes were registered.

We had expected to eat our tiffen at the station hotel in Tokyo, and take a train to Nikko, arriving in the evening; but we had no tiffin that day, or the next, or the next. Instead, all the afternoon of that day after the earthquake, we sat on the grass plot in the center of the plaza. There was plenty to see, but every moment we conjured up a vision of the earth opening, and grass plot, trees, and our puny selves disappearing.

A pile of grass mats, a short distance from where we were sitting, seemed to grow higher and higher each time I looked at them. Then I discovered that the mats covered the dead that were being collected from the wrecked buildings nearby.

Men were hurrying along with the old on their backs, some with bandaged arms and legs, all going as fast as possible in every direction. There was no screaming—no loud talking—no excitement of any description, a result of centuries of discipline.

Alice had remarked shortly after the first quake, "I have always heard that the most terrifying and disastrous happening in an earthquake is the fire that comes in its wake."

Tokyo was no exception! Only a few minutes after the quake, we saw smoke rising in the distance, and in one-half hour the Imperial University, just a few blocks away, was in flames.

All the afternoon we sat as idle as babies, with nowhere to go, nothing to do and nothing to do it with.

As evening impended, one of the Americans from the station hotel advised us, "Go to the park for the night; it's only a few blocks away, and will be quite safe." He brought us a blanket from the hotel, and a kettle of drinking water.

A school teacher from Iowa joined us, and we started for the park. But it was like finding a parking place in a busy city, for the park was already full of Japanese. We wormed our way through, and finally found enough space for the outspread blanket, on which we sat all night, at times dropping down on the ground for a wink of sleep.

The fires completely surrounded the park, and sometimes, almost obscured the sky leaving only a small patch above us. There was very little talking and absolutely no excitement. Here and there we saw and heard men carefully making their way through the squatting crowds of Japanese, calling for the lost. Melodious, unfamiliar names came mournfully through the air without disturbing me, for at that time I did not know that all the children in Tokyo of school age, had been wiped out in the holocaust of that day.

The first day of September, 1923, was the first day of school. The quake came just one minute before school was dismissed, and the children were trapped in the falling buildings, or caught in the fires. While in Tokyo I never saw a child of school age.

Our park companion, the Iowa teacher, was to have sailed the next day for Yokohama, on one of the President boats. She wore a thin muslin dress, with a light straw hat, and carried only a bead bag. She had come up to Tokyo just for the day, to visit some of its many fine schools. On her arrival she had taken a rickshaw to visit a school, when suddenly the boy stopped, snatched her out of the rickshaw, threw her face downward upon the ground, and placed his body over hers, supporting himself on his arms and knees. This terrified her more than the earthquake, but fortunately a man yelled, "Lie still. That boy is saving your life!" For four long minutes the buildings on each side came tumbling down. When it was over, the boy picked her up, dusted off her dress, put her back in the rickshaw, went straight to the station hotel, and left her so quickly that she never got an opportunity to pay him or even thank him.

When daylight came, after the weird Valkyrian night, we slowly picked our way back to the station hotel, to find that it had been threatened with fire, but that the wind had suddenly shifted, and it was still standing uninjured, without even a windowpane cracked, a victory for American steel and Frank Lloyd Wright's architecture.

Afraid to go into the hotel, we sat on the marble steps and listened to the stories of the destructive action of the earthquake in Yokohama, reported to be completely destroyed. One of the men at the hotel, an American who was in business in Yokohama, had come up to Tokyo just for the day, leaving his wife, quite an invalid, in the Grand Hotel, where they lived. His foot, injured by a falling brick, caused him to limp, but he never ceased trying to find someone who would go to Yokohama for news concerning his wife. Insane with anxiety as rumors of the destruction of Yokohama grew, he accosted everyone he met.

Immediately after the earthquake we had been put on rations, and everyone in Tokyo had for breakfast a cup of tea and a slice of bread; and for dinner, a bowl of broth with another slice of bread. Everyone was served, and all were served alike, but nothing was sold anywhere.

We spent the second night on the steps of the station hotel. "We" included a large group of Americans and English-speaking people. The American gentleman from Yokohama, who neither ate nor slept, told us he would watch and let us know if any danger threatened. Some slept, sitting up in chairs; some lay on the marble floor. All slept soundly till our watchman, who kept his eye on the chandelier hanging in the vestibule, screamed to us when it swayed to a right angle, "Go into the street!"

On the morning of the third day the American gentleman was relieved by getting news of his wife. One of the naval officers with whom he and his wife were very friendly, and who had been in the habit of spending evenings with them, was in a hotel a block away from the Grand when the quake began. He looked out of the window in his room, and saw only sky. Jumping out upon the window ledge, he slid down a waterspout and found his way to the Grand Hotel. Looking up to the windows of the rooms of his friends, he saw the wife of our companion standing naked in the window of her bathroom, where she had been in the tub when the quake started. Climbing to the bathroom window, the young officer pulled her through, and took her on his back to the ship, the Empress of Australia, where she was put to bed, and her arms and ribs, broken by her fall in the tub, cared for.

Then he started to walk to Tokyo to find the lady's husband, but he found the bridges out and buildings blocking the roads—a frightful journey! The husband was so grateful that he wanted to do something for the naval officer, who would not wait, for he wanted to hurry back to bring the wife news of her husband.

Since he could not be persuaded to remain, the American gentleman determined to get him a bicycle for his return trip. Finally, a young Japanese was found, who sold them his bicycle for $300 cash. The money was already paid, when suddenly the Japanese boy said, "No! No! My government might want it!" and pressed back the money.

At this juncture the American gentleman grabbed the boy around the waist and screamed to the naval officer, "Take it, and run like hell!" And when our clever gentleman limped into the hotel, he boasted, "Well, I begged a bicycle, I bought a bicycle, and finally, I had to steal a bicycle, but I got a bicycle."

One woman in our hotel-steps group had no milk for her baby, whereupon a Mr. Putney, who represented Little, Brown and Company, Boston, and an Irishman who had come down from Siberia to employ Japanese labor for his fisheries, volunteered to forage for milk. They walked and walked through burned districts, until they found shops in the sparsely settled regions beyond the fire. Picking up four bottles of milk, they started to pay the Japanese shopkeeper, but he shook his head, "No! no! not now."

As they started back to the hotel, a Japanese woman with a crying baby looked longingly at the milk, and the Irishman quickly gave her his two bottles. But the Bostonian put his in his pocket for fear of meeting more hungry babies.

Neither one of these men had had anything to eat for two days, and seeing a restaurant, they entered and ordered something to eat. They were served a good meal, but as they brought out their pocketbooks, the restaurant keeper shook his head. "No money! no money!" he insisted.

On the morning of the third day a Mr. Jonas, an Eurasian, accosted the hotel group. "I am going to try to reach Kobe, and if anyone wishes to join me, I will be glad to have him. It will be uncomfortable, and we may have to face danger."

We felt that, as we were already riding all four horses of the Apocalypse abreast, we should join the party. In all, there were fourteen: our group of four, a woman missionary returning to Shanghai, a Swiss artist, Mr. Putney, the Irishman from Siberia, Mr. Jonas, a Japanese man-servant, Mr. Jonas' brother-in-law, and three Japanese ladies.

All the automobiles and gas in Tokyo had been commandeered, but Mr. Jonas, on the plea of hurrying foreigners out of the city, was assigned one into which he loaded us all, with one small bag apiece. With policemen on the running boards to prevent our being injured by falling wires and tumbling walls, we rivaled the old woman who lived in a shoe.

We had not gone far when, afraid that the baking road and the stiflingly hot atmosphere of the still burning city might cause an explosion of the gasoline or the tires, we abandoned the automobile, joining the throng that filled the streets, all walking in the same direction in an attempt to escape from the city. Although everyone was calm and quiet, no one loitered.

After walking a couple of hours, we came to green grass, and then small villages. In the village streets were men and women with pails of water and drinking cups for the thirsty travelers. Our forced march came suddenly to a halt when Mr. Jonas announced, "The bridge has collapsed, and the people will have to cross in double file on a bridge of boats; so it will be a long time before our turn will come."

Thereupon, he conducted us to a nearby shed where we could wait, but on the way, the Swiss artist drew out of his pocket a bottle of liquor he had bought in one of the small villages. Mr. Putney, the missionary lady, the Irishman, Alice, and my cousin took a little, but Sarah and I refused.

This shed was empty, except for a platform on which my cousin made Alice lie down, take off her shoes, and have her feet rubbed. The missionary and the Irishman began to sing, and when Mr. Jonas arrived he found a gay party.

He had brought what food he could find—cans of lobster and pineapple, and boxes of animal crackers—not a balanced meal, but it tasted good to us, and was good for those who on an empty stomach, had taken too much out of the Swiss artist's bottle.

After eating we rested, but not long, for Mr. Jonas returned with news. "Our turn has come to cross the bridge of boats."

A bridge of boats—it took me back to high school Latin and Caesar—but when we landed on the other side, it was in a paddy field, and with every step we sank ankle-deep into the mud.

When at last we reached the railroad station, we found it to be the terminal of a short spur that linked up with the main line, and there were thousands of people ahead of us, waiting. We reached the station late in the afternoon, but it was midnight before we were able to board a train. There was no excitement, no one directing the crowds, no tickets, and no one pushing or taking undue advantage of his strength or opportunity. We walked about in the rain that had set in, or sat on the cinders which paved the ground, and watched the trains as they arrived, and the crowds that poured into them.

The men with babies in arms climbed upon the tops of the cars. The women were lifted through the windows until no more could be put in. Many clustered on the cowcatcher, and others filled the coalbox. When the train pulled out, it looked more like a huge caterpillar, than a train full of refugees.

When we were within boarding distance of the train, the crowds behind us were as large as the crowds had been ahead, when we had arrived hours before. In the train we sat three in a seat, and every inch of room in the aisles and platforms was full. Happily, it was not more than an hour before we reached the junction where we hoped to get a train on the main line.

As we left the car, Mr. Jonas said, "Now you can rest or do as you choose, but I will go to see when we can get away from here." We were out of the earthquake region with its incessant trembling beneath our feet, and in front of us, a perfectly good cement floor invited everyone to rest his weary body. We all stretched out, Swiss artist beside Japanese woman, Japanese servant next to missionary lady, next to me the Irishman from Siberia, and in no time, all of us were sleeping as we had not slept for four days.

It seemed too soon to be awakened when Mr. Jonas came to conduct us into the train yards, across innumerable tracks to a coach which he wishfully thought might be part of the train to be made up for Kobe. We waited an hour, and sure enough, Mr. Jonas was right—our coach was Kobe-bound. As we neared the loading platform, Mr. Jonas pointed to the waiting mob. "I advise you to crowd yourselves."

We huddled together, three in a seat, and the waiting throngs filled the coach, aisles, lavatories and platforms, until every inch of space was taken, and the train moved out to make instead of a twelve-hour, a thirty-six-hour trip to Kobe. On account of the damages due to the earthquake, we had to cross Japan, go down the western coast, and then recross to Kobe.

I have never enjoyed any trip so much as that good-luck, horseshoe-shaped journey over Japan. We quickly adjusted ourselves to riding three in a seat, for one would stand ten minutes, and then another take his turn, and I rather think it an improvement on ordinary train travel. We reached a town about every hour.

It was still very warm, and all the windows were wide open.

When the train stopped, we pinched ourselves lest we be dreaming, for all the car windows were filled with brown hands extending snow-white balls of rice, free for everyone. At the next town there were cups of mountain water and sandwiches for everyone, thrust through the windows by other brown hands. At another town came pears, and slices of bright yellow watermelon. As it was getting hotter, we hailed our next course—buckets of cracked ice and tiny bags of candy. The climax was reached about noon when a little bucket of water and a small clean towel were provided for each passenger. By this time we were so dirty and sticky that that dainty wash gave us a feeling of respectability and drove away our fatigue. This unique progressive luncheon was given by the Japanese Red Cross. We never opened our pocketbooks from the moment of the earthquake until we reached Kobe.

During that long ride, as a physician I became interested (the lavatory was filled with people) as to whether anyone was suffering from the deprivation. I asked Mr. Jonas to speak to the Japanese, and I asked the rest of our party whether they were uncomfortable, but it was a fact that the excitement, the lack of food and drink, and possibly the fear which all had suffered, had produced complete inhibition of the urinary secretion and intestinal peristalsis.

Reaching Kobe, we went to the hotel where we had stayed for one week when we first arrived in Japan. All the rooms were full, but the American proprietor gave up his office and put up a bed for Alice. The rest of us slept on futongs, heavy Japanese quilts spread on the stone floor of the porch just off the office where Alice slept.

On this long ride I was wearing rubbers, a pair of silk pajamas, a shirtwaist, and quite a splendid hat trimmed with lace. The missionary lady had looked very genteel and neat when we left Tokyo, but now the skirt of her dress was split from side to side across the back, and dragged along like a train behind her. When caught in the earthquake, Mr. Putney was wearing a thin silk suit. Yet, although he was able to buy some Japanese shirts in Kobe, the sleeves came only a little below his elbows. My cousin came to his rescue by cutting off the back tails of the shirts and splicing the sleeves to make them long enough.

The relief from impending danger gave us two happy, carefree weeks before the sailing of the Empress of Asia for home. That Alice had not collapsed on that journey from Tokyo to Kobe was a miracle. She had not walked for weeks on account of the serious intestinal infection in Peking, and was not prepared for roughing it for four days, with almost no food.

Not till we reached Kobe did we learn how severe the earthquake had been in Yokohama. The city had been completely demolished. The Grand Hotel, where we had stored our bags, and where we had actually contemplated a two-weeks' stay, had been literally swallowed up in the disaster, with one hundred and sixty-nine guests, many of them American. Only the American Express agent and a couple of coolies escaped from the building. As soon as the earthquake began, the American Express agent had vaulted over the counter in the lobby and escaped outside the building. His Japanese assistant started to leave by the counter gate, where the safe fell upon him, killing him instantly. When friends have extended sympathy for the loss of nearly all of our Chinese gifts and purchases, I have assured them that the greatest value in our property had not been destroyed. We had had the joy of receiving the gifts, the sport of bargaining, and the pleasure of selecting the goods we had bought. The most desirable articles we could replace, and as for customs, we might have been born en route.

This line of optimism brought from Alice, "Yes, Pollyanna, you have already convinced yourself that we have suffered no loss; instead, we have met with great good fortune."

I stood my ground. To make lemonade out of one's lemons is never impossible.

21

REPORTS ON TWILIGHT SLEEP AND MATERNAL HYGIENE

I HAD NO SPECIAL literary training in college and was such a poor speller that my letters entertained Alice as much as Josh Billings' funny spelling amused his readers of those days. Nevertheless, I had a desire to be more than one of the audience in medical society meetings, and my enthusiasm, especially over twilight sleep, led me very often to take up my pen.

In 1915, prompted by a desire to hasten the day when all women might be free from hours and sometimes days of agonizing childbirth pains, I wrote a book on scopolamine morphine anesthesia.

This was at the time of my greatest medical activity, when, if I was not busy with patients in my office, I was making house calls or operating and delivering babies in the hospital. In addition, I had regular hours for teaching and conducting a free clinic. Twilight sleep was then at the peak of its unpopularity. For that reason, instead of seeking a publisher I paid a printer to make the book for me.

When it was finally released, I placed it with the Chicago Medical Book Company, that promised to advertise it and in every way promote its sale. It was not a best seller, but as teaching does more for the teacher than the student, this book did more for the author than for the reader.

When I began the study of medicine, chloroform (first used in Scotland one year following the introduction of ether in the United States) was the popular anesthetic. But later, when chloroform was found to produce changes in the liver, harmful to health, and at times, to life, ether supplanted it, and for half a century has maintained its prestige, although during that period dozens of other anesthetics have made their debut.

The most recent anesthetics belong to a group of which scopolamine was the pioneer. Dr. Emil Ries, a skilled and progressive Chicago surgeon, was among the first to use it. I copied his method, and in my surgical clinic, where I found it safe and satisfactory for both my patients and myself, I used it routinely until I had a group of 5,000 operations done under this spectacular anesthetic. I think it spectacular, for after forty years' experience, I am still thrilled at seeing a patient brought to the operating room, unconscious of removal from her room, the ride on the rumbling cart, and the disagreeable preparation for operation. When the patient, back in bed, wakes up, she is surprised that the operation has been finished two to six hours before.

With the reported 5,000 cases of scopolamine morphine anesthesia, I included only one hundred cases of obstetrical anesthesia, for up to that time I held to the popular belief that scopolamine-morphine anesthesia was not good for the baby, and should be used with great care and caution in obstetrics. To enable me to use scopolamine, or, as it was popularly called, "twilight sleep," in the one hundred cases, the staff of the Women and Children's Hospital of Chicago very graciously turned over to me the obstetric service for one year. Following the instructions of Dr. Gauss of Germany, I administered twilight sleep routinely to all service cases in the hospital.

The first fifty cases both fascinated and disgusted me, for some patients would fall asleep after the first two doses, and be unconscious of their surroundings until after the baby was born, yet cooperate so that the baby could be born in a natural way. Others would scream, get out of bed, fight the nurses and interns, and on a few occasions climb out upon the fire escapes, and only with difficulty be induced to come back.

Although discouraged, we determined to try another fifty cases, but with different technique. Screens were made to fit around the beds: head, foot and sides. By passing a sheet of heavy canvas under the mattress, and up to the tops of the screens, we made a crib in which our twilight patient could lie.

The success of this crib labor bed was based on the fact that any pain continued too short a time for the patient, who was rather dazed, to climb over the top of the screen, or force her way out of the crib. As soon as this technique was introduced, the work and worry of the nurse was less than when caring for a patient without twilight sleep.

Another problem was to devise a delivery bed that would prevent the patient from disarranging the sterile sheets during the birth. We solved it by strapping the patient's knees into knee crutches constructed on the leg supports. With the help of these innovations the second fifty cases were so successful that the hospital continued the use of twilight sleep in obstetrics, and for the past twenty-five years their maternal and infant mortality has been among the lowest in this country.

The laity is always eager to learn about twilight sleep, but is confused by the older anesthetics (chloroform, ether, and gas) under the influence of which the patient is physically asleep, with her reflexes lost. That a patient can be absolutely unconscious of what is going on around her, and yet able to speak, move the arms and legs at will, and even bear down and give birth to a baby in the normal fashion, seems incredible. Twilight sleep is successful in childbirth because, by not inhibiting the reflexes, it does not lessen or suppress the contractions of the uterus, which are essential for the birth of the baby.

To watch a patient under the influence of scopolamine is both fascinating and enlightening. Dr. Vesper Shaffer, who had a very large and successful private obstetric practice in the northwestern part of Chicago, delivered hundreds of babies in the homes with the mothers under twilight sleep.

She described the behaviour of one of her patients. As soon as the labor began, Dr. Shaffer gave her the three initial doses of scopolamine, after which the patient was no longer conscious of her surroundings or her acts. When a pain came, she got out of bed and proceeded to make it up. Next she went into the kitchen, took the teakettle, filled it at the sink, and put it back on the stove. As the pains wore off, she returned to her bed and lay quietly resting till the next pain. Dr. Shaffer, in full view of the bed and the kitchen, saw the patient repeat these movements twenty times by actual count. As the patient was familiar with her own home, its furnishings and general arrangement, there was slight chance of her getting bewildered, and a crib bed, or any other form of restraint was unnecessary. Dr. Shaffer demonstrated, by the delivery of hundreds of cases in the home, the fallacy that twilight sleep could be used only in a hospital.

The employment of the reflexes to control the restlessness of patients under twilight sleep is important. In 1916, during a meeting of the American Medical Association in Detroit, I demonstrated twilight sleep in the Woman's Hospital. There were two patients in labor, one, an American woman trained in good manners, quiet and easy to manage under the anesthetic; the other a young, recently immigrated Russian woman. There were no crib beds, and the noise was distracting, for a dozen physicians were in each room, observing the labor and delivery. The American woman was ideal for demonstrating, and I was with her when I received an S.O.S. to come to the room where the Russian woman was laboring. I found her in the middle of the room, grasping a chair held high above her head, ready to crash down any minute. She was naked from the waist down, and three of the male visiting physicians were clinging desperately, but ineffectively, to her arms and legs. When I entered, I commanded everybody to leave the room except Dr. E. DeBlois whom I asked to stand with her back to the door. Picking up a sheet, I covered myself with it, leaving only my eyes exposed, and stood motionless. The patient dropped the chair, walked slowly and nonchalantly toward the window, looked out, and moved away towards the bed.

Thinking that a distended bladder had caused her excitement, I kicked a nearby pail, and in a loud voice called, "Here's the bucket." After contemplating the pail, she picked it up, went behind the bed, and relieved her bladder.

Taking advantage of the association between emptying the bladder and going to bed, I suggested again in a loud voice, "Get into bed." As twilight sleep patients are usually extremely modest, I added, "Someone is coming."

"Who?"

"A man."

At that, she jumped upon the bed, and covered herself up to her neck with the sheets.

Her reflexes proved to be most useful. Without them all the king's horses and all the king's men could never have put her into that bed, and left her calm and quiet.

The long period of unconsciousness produced by twilight sleep enabled me to develop a unique and successful technique in operating on toxic goiter.

Early in the morning the day following the patient's entrance into the hospital, I did a fake operation; that is, when the patient was deeply under twilight, she was taken to the operating room, where her neck was prepared and bandaged as it would have been if the operation had really been done.

When the patient wakened about noon, thinking the operation over, she and all her relatives (who were not in on the secret) were happy and relieved. At the end of the week when all active interest in the patient had subsided, without the knowledge of the patient or relatives, the real operation was done and the goiter removed. Waking and finding herself sitting up in bed, the patient was told that the dressings had been changed, but she did not know that the real operation had just been performed.

The nurses, always most loyal and cooperative, have never been found guilty of disclosing the facts either to patient or relatives. However, they are always surprised that patients are never suspicious, but after the fake often complain of pain in the incision, and inability to move the neck, and ask the nurse to hold and steady the head while they change its position.

The after-treatment of the fake operation is to keep the patient lying on her back with no pillow, and liquid diet for one week. After the real operation she is placed in a sitting position in bed, and put on a general diet. On the day of operation, a good meal is given and usually eaten.

The removal of fear, accomplished by twilight sleep, does more for the circulation than any medication or treatment.

Scopolamine has not only anesthetic, but also analgesic action (relief from pain) varying according to the dosage of the drug. Quite by accident I discovered its value in dental surgery.

After finishing a minor operation, I learned that my patient was very desirous of having all of her teeth removed. Curious to see if I could remove them under twilight, I did a thorough job, and the lady was not aware of her loss till hours afterwards, although during the extraction, she voluntarily had opened her mouth widely at my command and made no resistance. This experience in dental surgery stimulated me to renew my earlier accomplishments acquired at Kalamazoo. For tonsillectomy, combined with local anesthesia, scopolamine is superior to any other because it enables the patient to sleep for many hours after the operation.

In hospitals where the action of twilight sleep is not understood, and there are no crib beds or restraining delivery tables, twilight sleep makes great demands on nurses and interns as well as on obstetricians, and is justly unpopular.

At the Women and Children's Hospital of Chicago, nurses are taught that patients under twilight sleep should be handled as little as possible because efforts to force or restrain them cause excitement. Interns judge the progress of normal labor by watching the behavior of the patient who lies quietly or sleeps with only slight restlessness during a pain until the mouth of the womb is about half opened. Then she sits up during her pains until the mouth of the womb is completely dilated, when she squats tailor fashion on the bed and no longer lies down. If birth is imminent, she again lies down, usually on her side, and begins to bear down. The administration of ether to the twilight-sleep patient in labor is a serious mistake, even if forceps have to be used, because ether and chloroform paralyze the uterine muscles. Besides, the patient is already unconscious of her surroundings, and will remember no pain.

The administration of twilight sleep for surgery is quite different from that for obstetrics. In surgical operations it is imperative that the patient be absolutely quiet with reflexes abolished, and to insure this inhibition of the reflexes, morphine is combined with the scopolamine in each hypodermic dose. In childbirth, it is desirable that voluntary movements be preserved with active reflexes, to which end no morphine whatsoever is used. The standing order that no morphine or ether be administered, even at the end of delivery, may account for the infrequency of asphyxia at the Women and Children's Hospital. When scopolamine for childbirth anesthesia was first introduced by Kroenig and Gauss, it was combined with morphine, but the morphine has been gradually reduced, until, for the past fifteen years, no morphine has been used in our service.

The mental effect of twilight sleep on the mother is a blank. As a Negro woman who had this anesthesia expressed it, "Was that twilight sleep? To me, it was uttah darkness."

In surgical cases it is occasionally necessary to give a little ether, gas, or local anesthesia, in addition to the two or three doses of scopolamine and morphine, but I have operated on many, many cases, doing long, serious operations with scopolamine-morphine alone. The well-being that the patient experiences on waking is one of the happy advantages of twilight sleep, whether it be a surgical or an obstetrical patient.

Twilight sleep was under discussion at a medical meeting when Dr. Joseph De Lee asked Dr. Kurt E. Schloessingk of Freiburg, Germany, "What do you think about women who prefer to experience the pains, and object to an anesthetic?"

Dr. Schloessingk shrugged his shoulders, and extending his hands palms upwards, acquiesced, "If they vants to have their pains, let them have their pains."

Some men for lure of adventure go to the frozen regions of the poles to suffer and risk their lives, and no one should gainsay that privilege. If any woman has an urge to experience that great physical convulsion, childbirth, she should be allowed the privilege of being an observer, and if that has not satisfied her in full measure, she should, by all means, be encouraged to become acquainted with Nature in her most primitive of moods.

There are two schools in medicine: one believes that experiencing pain develops the emotions and strengthens the will; the other, that pain is an injury to the nervous system. I have been a witness to the truth of both pronouncements, but am convinced that the physician's continuous observation of unrelieved pain is more damaging to his sensibilities and spirit than the endurance of it to the patient's.

Midwifery exacts a toll of the mental, physical, and emotional reserves of the physician that is comparable to that in no other specialty, and for this reason, in solving the problem of obstetrical anesthesia, the obstetrician should be considered along with the expectant mother and the baby. For fifteen years after I began practice I delivered patients in their homes, and regardless of assistance it was I, the doctor, upon whom the morale of the patient and family rested. I was called when labor was evident, and I never left the patient until she had been delivered, whether it took hours or days. Many of my colleagues consider this a waste of time, but to me it is a practical application of the golden rule which I have found an unfailing solution to every problem I have ever met and fulfillment of my Hippocratic oath.

If I should leave the laboring woman with instructions to call me when she began to bear down or when the membranes ruptured, I would be unfit for any other professional work, for my mind would be filled with possible happenings to her whom I had deserted—the sudden development of a premature separation of the placenta—a rupture of the uterine wall—rupture of the membranes with prolapse of the cord—a precipitate labor with the patient alone and unprepared—no end of obstetric incidents that might cost one or two lives if I were not watchfully waiting at my post. Obstetricians are of two categories: one delivers the baby, the other attends the woman in labor.

Hospitalization of the obstetric patient decreases the time and inconvenience of the physician by seventy-five per cent. Hospitalization of patients of any class, and especially the obstetric, is an all-around saver of the doctor, but for me, obstetric twilight anesthesia is even more, because through it I am relieved of the job of morale-keeper; I catch up on my reading and writing; I am never harassed by relatives who want me to tell them things that are not even whispered in research laboratories; I am not worried lest the patient become exhausted; and although I am in constant attendance on the expectant mother under twilight sleep, she is only physically in the hospital—mentally she is in her peaceful home with all of its absorbing interests and familiarity. The isolation of the twilight-laboring woman in a hospital labor room gives the obstetrician complete control of everything, even her time.

The entry of the "man midwife" into obstetrics has been marked by great changes. The first and most important was the introduction of antisepsis by Semmilweis in 1847. The next advance was the turning of the baby in the womb, and effecting birth by traction on the baby's feet and legs. Before the obstetric forceps were introduced, this was the only way in which an unmutilated baby could be delivered in difficult labors. At the present time there are a number of male obstetricians who deliver all babies either by Caesarean section or by turning the baby. Either one of these methods places the delivery completely in the hands of the obstetrician.

One of our famous obstetricians has suggested that every mother be delivered of her first baby by forceps after the opening to the vagina has been cut. This method was given the name of "prophylactic forceps," and was not to be used by any physician except a specialist.

The increase in the operation of Caesarean section has been so great that it is now done on the slightest provocation, such as in a mother over forty with her first pregnancy. The operation requires less than an hour, and the mother is delivered free from all pain.

The most widespread innovation in modern obstetrics is the cutting of the muscles at the vaginal outlet. This goes under the name of "episiotomy" and is taught, advocated, and applied universally. The older midwives and obstetricians made an art of the slow and careful delivery of the baby's head without inflicting any injury to the muscles of the perineum at the outlet of the birth canal. Now no time is lost in allowing this beautiful natural process to take place, for the obstetrician assumes the responsibility for the time when the baby shall come, and the depth to which the mother shall be laid open to hurry the birth.

By instituting Caesarean section, version or turning of the baby, prophylactic forceps and episiotomy, the birth of a baby has been diverted from a delicate natural process, consuming hours, to short surgical procedure directly under the control of the operator.

With hospitalization and twilight sleep the road is open for a return of more physiological births. Obstetrics with twilight anesthesia is as different from obstetrics without that anesthesia as the world in peacetime from the world at war. Another advance in obstetrics, quite as important as twilight sleep, was the introduction of maternal hygiene. Besides saving the lives of many mothers and babies, it has also done much towards producing normal deliveries. I was impressed with the great interest on the part of the general public in the care of the expectant mother when I was assigned the responsibility of the production of a huge book six feet high and four feet wide. This book was designed as the central figure in a maternal hygiene exhibit in the Hall of Science at the Century of Progress in Chicago.

Medical women have always had to struggle for representation, and their part in the Century of Progress, as in the Columbian Exposition, was no exception to this rule.

In 1892, Chicago and the practice of medicine were so new to me that I was not even aware of the fight that medical women staged at that time for representation at the Columbian World's Fair. When Dr. Sarah Hackett Stevenson found out that medical women were to be allowed no part in that greatest of all fairs, she gathered her forces together and succeeded in getting a state appropriation for a Woman's Hospital exhibit. A building was erected in which the women doctors gave first aid and treated thousands of patients.

Forty years later, when arrangements for the Century of Progress were completed, the medical women were again excluded. In protestation, Dr. Lena Sadler and I appealed to the management for representation and space for some exhibit in the Hall of Science. We were told that, as there had been no arrangements for an exhibit on Maternal Hygiene, we might make an application for such an exhibit. However, there were a dozen applicants for the space, and if we wanted it, we would have to compete by presenting a perfect model of a maternal hygiene exhibit with all specifications. With the help of a hastily organized group of the medical, dental, and allied science women, we presented such a fascinating model that we were given the space.

The financing was more difficult—so difficult that Dr. Sadler and I found ourselves almost alone on the project. My democratic program was to collect one dollar from every medical, dental, and allied science woman in the United States, but Dr. Sadler said, "No, no. That's too long and hard a job. Go to Lane Bryant and ask them to allow you to exhibit their maternity dresses. I will go to Vanta, and then there's the Camp maternity corset. These firms ought to pay $500 for the privilege of exhibiting their products."

To my amazement, Dr. Sadler's plan brought us $6,000 in a few weeks so that the Medical, Dental, and Allied Science Women's Association for the Century of Progress was able to sponsor and furnish a booth on Maternal Hygiene in the Hall of Science, a booth on History of Women in Medicine in the

Hall of Social Science, and a booth devoted to Child Welfare on the Enchanted Island.

This huge book, that was to be the central feature in the Maternal Hygiene exhibit, was to have on one side of each page an oil painting of some feature in prenatal care, and on the opposite side, in hand-illuminated type, a question and answer explanatory of the picture. The management of the fifteen well-known artists who were to paint the pictures was my miserable job, and before the pictures were completed, I had exhausted all my diplomatic and dictatorial powers. Driving pigs, hiving bees, picking thorny blackberries, riding bareback, or teaching without sufficient preparation, were easy in comparison. I was, however, determined that the big book should draw the crowds and elevate the highest function of woman as well as the woman doctor.

The big book, especially the picture of an unborn baby and its technical advice to expectant mothers, was one of the most popular exhibits at the Fair and many people spent hours watching the woman physician hostess turn the pages and listening to her as she read the advice to expectant mothers.

In a small niche of that enormous building, the Rosenwald Museum of Science and Industry, this Maternal Hygiene Book is safely guarded and is waiting for the day when it will be installed in the Medical Women's Library and Memorial Hall on the campus of the Woman's Medical College of Pennsylvania.

MANY ROADS TO HEAVEN

DR. GUNSAULUS, dean of the Armour Institute in Chicago, and a celebrated divine who filled the four thousand seats in the Auditorium every Sunday, once remarked, "Our friend, Miss Bullard, and I always agree. She is an orthodox-liberal, and I am a liberal orthodox."

Turning to me, he catechised, "What art thou?"

"Well," I replied, "I will leave it to you—last week, on Sunday, I baptized an unborn child of Catholic parents because its life was in danger. On Wednesday, I was the only woman attending a Jewish circumcision, the parents refusing to have the mohel operate without my presence—on Friday, with a tiny casket in my arms, I went alone to the cemetery with the body of a baby whose parents did not believe in funerals."

Dr. Gunsaulus grasped my hand.

22

MURDER?

I WAS in the Women and Children's Hospital at seven o'clock in the morning of November 23, 1933, when I read and reread, then slowly spelled out the big black letters in the headline, "Rheta Wynekoop Murdered."

My early operation was, for the time, forgotten as I concentrated my thoughts on who could have committed such a crime. I was sure that it must have been some irresponsible crazy person. At that moment any idea that Dr. Lindsay Wynekoop might have murdered Rheta, would have been as untenable and fantastic as a suspicion against me.

Rheta was the beautiful, delicate wife of Dr. Wynekoop's son, Earl. Ever since their marriage a few years before, the young couple had lived with Dr. Wynekoop who not only admired but loved her daughter-in-law. She was always arranging appointments for Rheta, a fine violinist, to appear on programs.

Shortly after Rheta became one of the family, Dr. Frank Wynekoop and the adopted daughter died and Rheta seemed to make up in many ways for their losses.

My friendship for Dr. Lindsay Wynekoop began when she was a medical student. Of decided beauty and charm, her head covered by masses of wonderful titian hair that curled about her face, Miss Lindsay lit up and made beautiful everything about her, even her clothes. I was very happy when, five years after her graduation, she married Dr. Frank Wynekoop who had devoted much of his time to me and given me, without remuneration, the instruction necessary to teach embryology.

Their first child was a beautiful boy named Lindsay. When but a baby, he died following an attack of appendicitis. Dr. Lindsay Wynekoop took the death badly; in fact, her three later children never quite took the place of the boy Lindsay. Walker, her second son, was a lusty, handsome little fellow of great promise.

Unfortunately, Dr. Lindsay Wynekoop's health was never robust. I saw her one day in front of a big department store downtown in Chicago, where she had been having a severe pulmonary hemorrhage. Hence, although she recovered, it was no shock to her friends when, with her fourth child, Earl, husband of Rheta, she kept persistently to her bed nearly the whole prenatal period, to prevent losing him. As it was, he was born prematurely, and proved a difficult baby to rear. Feeling a certain responsibility for his prematurity, she always gave him a little more care, a little more consideration and more shielding from any ills, than the other children.

Passionately fond of babies, she would sacrifice herself for children and young people, hers or someone else's, as she looked after the smallest needs of her little family. After the birth of her daughter, who was vigorous like the older brother, Dr. Wynekoop, undaunted by the care of three children, adopted a little girl, Mary Louise, in order that her own small daughter might have the companionship of a sister.

It was a busy, happy family during those years while the children were growing up. In a small room off the dining room, the four children ate their meals. The cute little table, the tiny chairs, the cunning dishes, and the pretty, appropriate pictures on the wall must certainly have done much to make those childhood days of the Wynekoop children unforgettable. Great care was given to their schooling; each child was studied and placed where it could develop in the most normal way.

Dr. Wynekoop, although her father was an atheist, was herself a most devout Episcopalian. She confided one day that she went to her pastor for confession, an institution that she believed to be of great help.

Dr. Frank, her husband, was a quiet man, like a boy who had been brought up in the country and had never gotten far away from country habits and country thinking. Deeply interested in medical science, had he been engaged in research instead of general practice, he would probably have made some important scientific discovery.

Inasmuch as a nucleus of devoted patients had grown year by year into a large and lucrative general practice, they always had funds to keep the children looking lovely, and to give them every advantage of children of wealth.

Almost daily we talked over the telephone. It mattered little whether it was Dr. Lindsay or Dr. Frank that I got first; I always had a delightful chat with each one. I enjoy a gay companion, and of all the friends I have ever had, there was never any gayer than she. Even in serious things she saw something amusing, and met every light vein of mine with peals of laughter, so sudden, loud, and irrepressible that it seemed beyond her control. I sometimes wonder if her close and constant association with her children kept her so young and mirthful.

It was, however, through her patients sent to me for operation, that I found how generous and unmercenary she was. She would often say, "Now, my services are not worth anything, but I want you to know what hard times this patient has been having." Then she would finish a hard-hit story by begging, "Do make your charges small!" Occasionally she would say, "Could you do the operation for nothing?"

In 1934, only a few months after her commitment to the Reformatory at Dwight, I gave voice in a toast to my feelings about Dr. Alice Wynekoop at a dinner given during the American Medical Association meeting in Cleveland. It was in honor of Dr. Rosalie Slaughter Morton, who was presented with a loving cup by some of her friends. Dr. Emily Barringer of New York

City, toastmistress, had asked me to respond to a toast but gave no hint as to what she would like me to say. My crony, Dr. Lena Sadler, was then president of the American Medical Women's Association, and when I began to tell her what I had intended to say at the dinner, she protested, "No! no! Just get up, say a few graceful words, and sit down. Promise me you will."

For some reason my mind seemed to run amuck. I had never before thought of so many wonderful speeches I could make but I valued my dear friend Lena's advice. She was wise and sane, and I knew I ought to obey. I would have, if I could have spoken first.

But I thought and thought all through the dinner as I sat in front of the large loving cup. The first one called upon for a toast was the only male present—a gentleman who eulogized and emphasized the "lady doctor," the "woman physician," the "fair sex," the "lovely lady" . . . .

I offer this as a feeble excuse for my wretched toast, so quizzically received. I rose, and looking straight over Lena Sadler's head, ignoring her in fact, I began with, "I know exactly how proud and happy this occasion and this loving cup make my friend, Dr. Morton. I know, because once upon a time, after I had been practicing medicine for twenty-five years, a very dear friend of mine arranged for me just such a dinner; and she, too, bought a loving cup on which were engraved the names of all of my women doctor friends on the hospital staff. I was so proud and happy that I placed the loving cup upon the mantel where its beauty could inspire me every day with the love and loyalty of my friends.

"Well, the days went by and the years rolled over, and I know not why, but it happened that my loving-cup friends put me off the hospital staff, and I took down the cup. I spat into it, and relegated it to the attic, to collect rust and dust, to be observed by mice, not men.

"The days went by and the years rolled over, and I know not why, but it happened that my loving-cup friends begged me to go back on the hospital staff, and I went groping into the attic, and found the loving cup. After much polishing it did look pretty, and I could read all the names that had been dimmed by the dust and dirt. I was glad to go back to the hospital, and I restored the loving cup to its place of honor on the mantel.

"And the days went by, and the years rolled over, and I cannot see why, but it happened that the dear one who had bought the loving cup for me so long ago, was accused of murder and committed to prison, where she is now languishing. My first impulse was to take the cup from off the mantel, roll it in cotton and hide it away, never to take it out until she was vindicated and restored to honor.

"Now, I am telling this to Dr. Morton that she may know in advance that loving cups may be full of love, or they may be full of gall and bitterness; but my wish is that hers will let everything, except love, leak through."

When Dr. Morton spoke, I caught Dr. Sadler's eye. It was ominous with that look of "Mother will have to spank."

The loving-cup dinner, arranged by Dr. Alice Wynekoop, was her first effort to bring my friends to a happy recognition of me. Her next attempt in that direction was a very successful and never-to-be-forgotten occasion, a Farewell Dinner as she called it, on the eve of my departure for China in 1922. The dinner was given at a Greek restaurant on Ogden Avenue, midway between Cook County Hospital and the medical school, because Dr. Wynekoop thought that I would feel more at home in surroundings that were part of my daily medical routine.

Dr. Quine, Dean of the University of Illinois College of Medicine, and his niece were there. Dr. Quine was acknowledged to be the most eloquent and moving of speakers; he never was more so than on that evening. He had a fatherly pride in my going to China to lend my assistance in every way possible to many women medical students whom I had helped to prepare for their mission work.

At this Farewell Dinner Dr. Wynekoop had a speaker to represent each group and society or club of which I was, or had been, a member. The program was really ingenious.

There were clever innovations that no one but Dr. Wynekoop could have conceived. She called upon Dr. Margaret Jones to respond to a toast for the "Society of Redheads." Dr. Jones, Dr. Wynekoop and I were all brilliant specimens of that society.

At that time I had literally tons of copper-yellow hair. It was so thick and long, reaching to my knees, that I could dispose of it in no other way than by braiding it into two huge braids and winding them about my head, like a cap. I had always entertained an intense hatred of this hair, and no amount of praise could convert me.

As a child I had been "Redhead," "Sorreltop," "Carrots," and all the red-hot names country children can conjure up. As a young lady, I had worn my hair in only one style and never in the prevailing fashion. As a surgeon, I had spent time and money having it shampooed and cleaned for the aseptic technique of the operating room. When finally it turned grey, and fashion demanded that it be bobbed, I was as happy as a boy with a rabbit. I would look into the mirror, and at times feel a little ashamed that at long last I could see something in my reflection to excite my admiration, for to me, my grey bobbed hair was a perfect success.

The program was terminated by calling upon Dr. Julia Holmes Smith, pioneer woman physician and ex-president of the Chicago Woman's Club, to give a prayer. That prayer still rings in my ears, so simple, so full of fervor.

This Farewell Dinner was a sweet, intimate affair in comparison with a banquet that Dr. Wynekoop conceived and executed ten years later on the event of my seventieth birthday. She called this banquet an Appreciation Dinner, and mustered to it such a distinguished group of people that it was I who felt cheap and small, almost shoddy, to be having so much attention from the elite of the profession, as well as from shining figures in social and political life.

Again as toastmistress, Dr. Wynekoop inspired the guests to outdo each other in a rivalry of praise and appreciation.

Alice was unable to attend the dinner, but she wrote me a

letter. That letter I prize more than any of the things said about me that night:

> My precious sister,
> People will say all sorts of lovely things to you and about you tonight, but they will not know as I do how true they are. Accept this tribute from one who has leaned on your loyalty, been strengthened by your love, been happy always by the sunshine of your optimism, who is most thankful for your existence.

The confidence Dr. Wynekoop and I placed in each other was impregnable. If at that Appreciation Dinner any one had told me that in less than a year she would be serving a twenty-five year sentence for the murder of her daughter-in-law I would have been positive that either one or both of us had lost our sanity.

During those bleak months of November and December when, printed in bold type, the headlines revealed every day some fresh circumstantial evidence against Dr. Wynekoop, I was certain that she was not guilty. Day after day and night after night I strove to collect irrefutable proof of her innocence.

Through the weakness of sick bodies and the urge of sore conscience the physician often comes into possession of a fund of information—secrets that she must keep as Nature keeps her secrets, and never divulge; others may find them out only by their own investigations.

A remark, a confidence, a promise, a fact, a story, the history of a patient, the mutterings of one anesthetized, the ravings of a maniac, if blended and brewed like the ingredients of a good recipe, may come to form the solution of a knotty problem.

Along such lines and out of such material, step by step, I developed the theory substantiated with proven facts and common sense, that Rheta Wynekoop was not murdered, but accidently shot, although fatally, by an irresponsible person.

The next step was to get this story into the trial already underway. I have no aptitude for law and was soon made to realize that by pushing my murder theory I might be obstructing the case already set up for her defense. Disappointing as were my efforts during the trial, after the verdict they were hopeless.

During the fifty years of my friendship with Dr. Lindsay Wynekoop, a big opportunity to demonstrate my deep love for her never came until the middle of December, 1943, when she telegraphed me to come at once to the Reformatory at Dwight, Illinois.

This is the only time Dr. Wynekoop telegraphed me, but I have received many letters from her. One especially gives the daily routine of her prison life. Her days are all alike:

> My old pal! Could I but grip your hand and sit where I could see you awhile. I'd not need many words! Times I feel as though I'd literally succumbed to the desperate need of someone who *cares*. All my life, until imprisoned, there were those within touch or call who satisfied this deep need. Just can't seem to get along without it. My schedule is pretty well defined: called at 6:30, breakfast at 7:00, "do" my room and report for assignment, 7:45. Back in room 11:40, shower and change work suit for dress and dinner 12:00. In my room again (with door locked) until 12:30. Then until 1:15 am enjoying a bit of tutoring for someone who has a laudable ambition—I like doing that! At 1:15 I go to the solarium, where I rest an hour; then until 4:45 read and brief (for filing) selected medical articles. Supper is at 5:30; lights out at 8:30... For "pickup" an undertaking lace for an altar cloth. It is No. 50 thread so that I cannot do more than fifteen minutes at a time. It is hard, but am making it a devotional service. All that time I'm at prayer...

On my arrival at the reformatory I was conducted to a pleasant room to meet the doctor who was with one of the parole officers, a delightful lady, not at all like a prison guard. On previous visits I had seen her in the visitors' basement waiting room, where we sat at a long table with a high glass partition separating us, and a grim female "matronizing." Often I had to wait an hour to see her, and our time was always limited to visiting hours.

Dr. Wynekoop had sent for me to advise her regarding her petition that would come up before the Division of Pardons and

Paroles on January 11, 1944. She talked rapidly, referring to notes, and was in every way a different Dr. Wynekoop from the one I had grown used to—the despairing, helpless prisoner. Her whole being was surcharged with determination and directness. I remarked on her changed attitude, and she confessed to a new outlook.

"When the doctor told me in September that there was a tiny spot on my lung, I suddenly made up my mind that, if I should have a return of the tubercular trouble that I had when a girl, I was not going to die here. It's strange, perhaps, but true that for ten years I have daily expected the real murderer to confess and exonerate me. Now I have given up that idea, and I am going to get out of here. I will! No matter what it costs—publicity, anything—I have stayed here long enough."

She had made out a list of old friends, whom she hoped still might be interested enough to help her. Her last request was that I should appear before the Board of Pardons in Springfield, Illinois, and make a thirty-minute plea.

The longed-for big opportunity to serve her had come, but it took my breath away! Although numberless times, to small groups of women or individuals interested in the case, I had detailed the circumstances that led (I believed) to the accidental shooting of Rheta Wynekoop by an irresponsible, or perhaps insane person, was I after all, the best one for such a responsible undertaking? My heart was full of resentment against her unjust imprisonment. My tongue tingled with hot, acid words. How unhappy I would be if, by some blazing word of wrath, I should cement, instead of sunder the shackles that, every year for ten long years, have sunk deeper into her sensitive soul. On the other hand, if I could rouse and touch human sympathy for her by my pleas, how happy I should be!

Whether for better or for worse, if she wished me to make a plea, I could not refuse her. She, more than any other friend, had a right to ask me to lay my heart upon the block, if need be, and do it as a happy sacrifice. In such a spirit I took upon myself my greatest responsibility in eighty years.

What I most needed was the advice that Alice and Sarah would give me. I also needed the quiet isolation of the farm, and so planned to spend the holidays in Stony Creek. To ease my conscience regarding travel in war time, I rode all night in a coach filled with soldier and sailor boys, women with babies, and sweethearts of every description, and arrived at the only place I call home, the day before Christmas.

To read a paper or speech always fills me with "stage fright"; I make a more pleasant impression upon my audience by extemporizing, assisted by a few notes. For this occasion I was determined to write and then commit to memory, my plea. However, I did not find writing easy. Day after day I wrote—and destroyed what I had written.

I wanted the gentlemen on the Pardon Board to understand that my friend was no common person, but a medical woman of parts and certainly not a murderer. For that reason I wrote in detail her medical and social attainments:

In 1893 she was a student in the Northwestern University Women's Medical School, where I was teaching embryology. During her senior year she began teaching in her Alma Mater and continued after graduating, first as Instructor of Anatomy, and later as chief demonstrator in the dissecting room and Clinical Assistant to Dr. D. R. Brower, specialist in nervous and mental diseases. In 1896 she interned in the Women and Children's Hospital. During the summer months of the years of 1897 to 1902 she was Resident Physician at the Daily News Fresh Air Fund Sanitarium. After her marriage to Dr. Frank Wynekoop in 1900, she became instructor in Histology at the University of Illinois College of Medicine and held this position from 1900 to 1914.

Besides these heavy rounds of medical work she took part in cultural, educational and philanthropic projects.

For two years she was President of the Chicago Medical Women's Club, and for another two years served as Chairman of the Propaganda Committee of the Chicago Medical Society, and presided at weekly lectures in the Chicago Public Library.

She was member and one of the three Trustees of the National Chapter of Nu Sigma Phi. She was a member and for a number of years acted as Corresponding Secretary of the Chicago Eugenic Education Society. In 1912 she was Chairman of "Baby Week," and conducted daily morning and afternoon clinics at the Boston Store in Chicago.

During World War I she was tireless in her efforts to disseminate knowledge regarding Social Hygiene and First Aid. She was a member of the Social Hygiene Committee of the Women's Division National Council of Defense, and a lecturer on Social Hygiene in Illinois, Indiana, Michigan and Wisconsin, under the auspices of the National Y.W.C.A. She served also at this time as Director of First Aid under the Red Cross.

She was a member of the Child Welfare Committee of the Woman's City Club, member of the Board of the Chicago Culture Club, Children's Benefit League, Chicago Political Equality League and the Illinois Congress of Mothers, later known as the P.T.A., in which organization she has a life membership.

She was a charter member of the Cordon Club.

For several years she served as President of The West End Mother's Council and often as Chairman of the Program Committee. She was Director of Mothers' Classes at the Off the Street Club for many years, and for a short time taught an adolescent class in Epiphany Sunday School.

In this draft of my speech I only cautiously referred to the accidental shooting—my theory of the murder of Rheta—but stressed Dr. Lindsay Wynekoop's treatment during the "examination" made by the police. I told of the grilling, when she was allowed no rest, no change of clothing, no meals except a cup of coffee, when collapse seemed iminent. Even a visit to the lavatory, where there was no soap, towel or toilet paper, was made under male police escort.

During this "third degree" Dr. Wynekoop was taken from one police station to another. Entrance was difficult because of a mob, both men and women, who swarmed about them, cursing, calling vile names and spitting on her. These men and women did not know Dr. Wynekoop—had never seen her before. In three days, printers' ink had blotched out her life-long good name and branded her a murderer.

The press really tried Dr. Wynekoop. Every day she was hypothetically connected with some known crime. She was represented in pictures as an old hag plotting the death of anyone who came within her influence. Nor was it a matter of purely local interest. Every newspaper in the United States vied with those of Chicago in tearing her reputation into shreds. As her reputation shrank the coffers of the public press bulged.

This terrible impression made on the public by the press was not transient. Just recently a patient told me that she had never seen or known Dr. Lindsay Wynekoop, but she was quite sure that she was a vicious woman. She remembered how she had run a "baby farm," had murdered her husband, and she thought that she had put the body of her adopted daughter into the furnace.

The stimulus for this interest and wide-spread publicity was, without doubt, to be found in the fact that Dr. Wynekoop was a woman doctor, one of a group that has suffered long years from prejudice. When Dr. Elizabeth Blackwell was studying medicine almost a century ago, women who met her on the street would draw aside their skirts, lest they brush against such a bold, unwomanly creature. Dr. Wynekoop had unwittingly stirred up old smoldering fires of discrimination, and they burned with unquenchable ferocity.

Dr. Lindsay Wynekoop had hosts of friends, for the most part women, but they seemed powerless to help her.

When I read this plea that I thought was fairly strong to Alice she said, "I thought you wanted to free Dr. Wynekoop! Don't you? Or would you rather vent your spleen against the press and air your feministic views?"

I was now sure that I was not the person to make an effective plea, and I had only ten days in which to try to "change my spots." I wrote a new plea, cutting out the Who's Who, for I recalled that it was written out in full in the petition. I toned down, and smoothed out the activity of the press.

My next step on my return to Chicago, was to submit a typewritten copy of the much revised plea to Pearl Hart, one of Chicago's leading lawyers. After a careful reading, she advised me to delete some ungracious remarks about Dr. Wynekoop's lawyers, but urged that I enlarge upon my murder theory—give all names, places and dates in detail. She assured me that I need not fear doing so, for I had a right to my theory, and a right to make it public. She also suggested that as the Pardon Board was made up of men, it might be desirable to omit anything that might irritate them.

For ten years I had longed to cry from the housetops that Rheta Wynekoop was not murdered, but was accidently shot by an insane person. In no court had I ever been able to tell this, but before the Board of Pardons—yes! At last I was sure of my ground, and made the final draft of my plea with no difficulty.

On the morning of January 11, 1944, I made a forty-minute speech for the pardon of Dr. Lindsay Wynekoop after the Chairman of the Board had directed me, "Make your speech."

The plea that I made on January 11, 1944, in re the pardon of Dr. Alice Lois Lindsay Wynekoop follows:

Members of the Division of Pardons and Paroles
Springfield, Illinois
Gentlemen:

In petitioning for the pardon of Dr. Alice Lindsay Wynekoop, two typewritten pages were required to record her medical and social prowess, and it is, therefore, not necessary for me to review them. Few medical women, in double the number of years, have acquired recognition in as many fields—medicine, education and philanthropy.

My acquaintance with Alice Lindsay began in 1893, a half century ago, when she was a student in the Northwestern University Woman's Medical School where I was teaching embryology.

In 1900 she married Dr. Frank Wynekoop, a good friend to me, and in the past fifty years the Wynekoop family has been

Her entire family, from the nearest to the most remote member, was branded with the ever-active stigma of disgrace.

Dr. Lindsay Wynekoop was not only sentenced to twenty-five years' imprisonment, but like a guilty soldier from whom all insignia have been ruthlessly torn, she was stripped, in public, of all her hard-earned decorations: reputation, license to practice, membership privileges, and citizenship.

Dr. Lindsay Wynekoop, an innocent woman, has spent ten years imprisoned in the State Reformatory for Women at Dwight, Illinois, where she has performed every kind of labor for which she was physically able. She has worn the clothing, kept the hours, eaten the food, and lived up to the rules of the institution. She has accepted the limitations regarding visitors and correspondence. She has given freely of help and sympathy to her fellow prisoners. She has kept her mind young by reading current literature, the daily newspapers, medical journals and all the books and papers that thoughtful friends have sent to her.

In these ten long, monotonous years her Bible has been her solace, and prayer, that gives her strength, is ever on her lips and in her heart.

In 1937 I visited an old friend and patient who, at the age of thirty-five, forsook her life of teaching and residence in busy, bustling Chicago, to enter a cloistered convent, an hour's ride from London, England. On my return home I went to the State Reformatory at Dwight to see Dr. Lindsay Wynekoop, and was struck by the similarity of the lives of those two friends.

Convent walls keep the world from the cloistered nun, while prison walls keep Dr. Wynekoop from the world. The nun is restrained by vows and her duress is voluntary. Dr. Wynekoop's duress is compulsory and her restraint, the law. Nevertheless, the life of the cloistered nun is no more consecrated to the service of our Lord than the life of Dr. Lindsay Wynekoop.

Although Dr. Lindsay Wynekoop has petitioned for a pardon, she does not expect the State of Illinois to restore her reputation, for under the shadow of her lost reputation, her character, which no law or court can take away, has grown strong and enduring. She does not ask for a renewal of her right to practice medicine, for time, year by year, is making it null and void.

She does not seek reinstatement of her membership in the many medical and social organizations to which she belonged, for physical disability bars participation, except in memory.

She does not miss the loss of franchise, for, by reason of her sex, she had no vote until she was forty years of age. She is accustomed to such handicaps.

Dr. Lindsay Wynekoop petitions his Excellency, the Governor of Illinois, for her liberty, in order that the medical profession, all women, her sorority sisters, members of all the organizations to which she has belonged, her church, her friends, and most of all her family, may be spared the humiliation of having one of their number, though innocent, die within prison walls.

In every corner of the world young men are fighting and dying, that we may live in freedom. In a little corner of no man's land an old woman is fighting to live, and living in the hope that she may die in freedom.

Members of the Division of Pardons and Paroles:

I thank you for listening to my plea for the liberty of Dr. Lindsay Wynekoop. Because I know that she is innocent of her daughter-in-law's death, and had no part in it, her incarceration for a longer time demands great consideration and study. My words are but a poor sample of what is in my heart. In making recommendation for her pardon, I sincerely pray that you may have Divine Guidance and the inspiration of the Golden Rule, "All things whatsoever ye would that men should do to you, do ye even so to them." More than that no man can ask.

Though my plea brought some of the members of the Pardon Board to the verge of tears, nevertheless, Dr. Wynekoop was not granted a pardon. I did not know at this time that the board of pardons had received 31 petitions for pardons, and I had forgotten an impending election.

I did not mention in my plea the confession that she signed

three days after her arrest because she immediately repudiated it. Her signature was obtained after she had been falsely told that her son, Earl, was in the next room writing a confession.

The day following the plea, on January 11, 1944, Dr. Lindsay Wynekoop wrote me. The last paragraph of her letter gives her unalterable attitude towards her incarceration, as well as to her pardon:

> How will all this terminate? It is now in God's hands. May the work done in His name have response conformatory to His will. Since petitions (yours, Father Hopkins', all friends' and mine) have been *only for justice,* then we have in reality asked only 'Thy will be done,' God grant it.

I was glad that Dr. Wynekoop could rest her case with the Lord.

For myself, I swore, "I'll make them hunt their holes! I'll let them know there's a God in Israel!"

THE CUCKOO CLOCK

WHEN ON THE farm, I am often wakened in the night by the little bird in the cuckoo clock that rolls out the quarter hours in a sociable way, and am reminded of the patient who brought me in one year the thrill of victory and the devastating grief of failure. The patient had had only one child, and was so desirous of another that I operated on her, removing a parasitic fibroid tumor that had no attachments, nourished simply through numerous adhesions. These adhesions involved the diseased tubes and ovaries, and when the operation was finished, the patient was left with only a half-inch of Fallopian tube on one side, and a pinch of ovary on the other. I was excited when under such conditions she became pregnant. After a normal pregnancy I delivered her of a large, well-formed baby boy.

To express their gratitude the parents purchased the largest cuckoo clock they could find. I had always desired one; and there were no happier people than the parents and I, till one day I noticed that the baby's tongue protruded from its mouth —I could not bear to think of it—like a Mongolian idiot's. When I could not deny the diagnosis, I told the parents. Looking upon me as God must have looked upon Eve when she destroyed His Paradise, they led me to the front door and said, "Never enter this house again." Two months later I was gladdened to hear that the baby had died of pneumonia. My heart still grieves for this couple, but often I have told this story to console a patient who has been disappointed in her highest hopes by having a miscarriage.

23

SHANGRI LA

IF ALICE'S TALENT for home building had been directed into commercial channels, she would have been the financial victress in the family. Her efforts, begun in youth, have continued throughout her life. She has transformed house after house into a place of unbelievable charm, for like primitive woman she was endowed with the magic to convert, out of simple materials close at hand, comfort, convenience and beauty.

Though she preferred city life, and had never cared for the farm, when Sarah entered upon her career as a farmer I knew that Alice and I should build the remnants of our future around Sarah, with a home for all of us in Stony Creek.

In 1921, the year that Sarah took her Ph.D. degree, we made a start by setting out fruit trees and building a stone wall around the immense lot on which Grandfather had erected the farmhouse, one hundred years before.

During 1924, 1925, and 1926, our Stony Creek village workmen completed the house which is a visible expression of Alice's genius for homemaking.

Here garden lovers linger at any time of the year. The devotee of antiques finds grazing ground. The collector of travel souvenirs is fascinated by rare bits. Admirers of large rooms, quaint nooks, story-and-a-half beamed ceilings, low French doors and windows, great fireplaces, balconies, curved stairways and high wood wainscoting, find them here. There is nothing representing a great outlay of money, for simplicity is Alice's slogan.

Undoubtedly this attractive home is helpful to Sarah's farming business. To Alice it is a realization of her heart's desire—a dream come true. But to me, it is my Shangri La—the place where, by passing from room to room, I revitalize experiences that have come to a country-born woman who for fifty years has poured her energies into the cast of a medical career.

In the library hangs a beautiful oil painting of a canal in Venice. It brings back delightful days that I spent in Venice, but more than that, it recalls a serious hysterectomy that I performed on the wife of the artist who painted the canvas. She had been my sorority sister in Ann Arbor, but after her marriage and the birth of her only son, lived an invalided life for fifteen years. When I saw her as a patient, she requested, "I wish you would treat me as though I were a poor patient in the stockyard district." She referred to radical treatment. After her operation she made a satisfactory recovery.

Hanging opposite is an oil portrait of Hannah Olson, dressed in her mother's gay Swedish wedding garments. Hannah came to us as maid of all work, and proved to be a perfect housekeeper and cook. She had been with us two years when she surprised me by announcing that it had been her life's ambition to become a midwife, and no argument could dissuade her. After becoming a licensed midwife, and practicing in a Swedish community in Chicago for a couple of years, she again astounded me by returning and begging to be reinstated as our maid. She confessed, "I despise the class of people who employ midwives, and I would rather work in your kitchen."

I told her, "You must not come back as our maid; you were always too big for your job. I want you to take a course in a nurses' training school."

This time she accepted my advice and entered Tabitha Hospital Training School for Nurses, where she was given a year's credit for her proficiency in midwifery and housekeeping. As soon as she graduated, Hannah and I started what might be called a suburban midwifery service. I gave the prenatal care in my city office, and when the expectant mother was within two weeks of her time for delivery, Hannah was sent to the patient's suburban residence to prepare for the home delivery, assist the patient in taking her baths, care for her breasts, and attend to her diet. When labor began, Hannah notified me, and as soon as the delivery could be prognosticated, I joined her. After delivery I was able to leave the patient at once, never making more than one or two post-partum calls.

This delightful suburban midwifery practice was kept up for more than ten years, at the end of which time Hannah married and moved to western Canada, while I began to hospitalize all obstetrical patients. For patient, nurse and physician, this suburban practice was perfect. Yet I recognized that there was but one Hannah and that I was an exception in not regarding distance as an obstacle.

Musical chromosomes have been distributed as condiments rather than a *piece de resistance* in the Taylor and Van Hoosen family. No one of them has ever shown talent in music, yet we all enjoy a little of certain kinds. Father thought a piano was impractical and expensive, and often said he did not want his girls to be "little music teachers." Therefore, a piano was never a part of our parlor furniture until, after I had been practicing several years, I came in a most unusual way into possession of a walnut-cased Mathushek.

One morning at four o'clock my doorbell was rung by a patient who belonged to the world of clandestine sports, and she lay bare her predicament. "This morning the officers are coming to take my furniture. I don't care about any of it except my piano. I noticed you didn't have one—will you take mine? If you never see me again, it is yours."

Before five o'clock that morning the piano arrived, and since that time I have never seen the patient. But the piano is now in the library, where I enjoy it just as illiterate people enjoy the possession of handsomely bound books. The character of its owner never disturbs me, for people who lead lives screened from the law or the world of convention possess a more lively sense of justice, more of that brother's-keeper feeling and more loyalty than I have ever discovered in persons ostentatiously united to refound the earth. I have often chanced upon this honor among thieves.

Though not connected with it, the piano always suggests to me a tragic story. One of my patients, living in a handsome way on Grand Boulevard, was the ravishingly beautiful wife of a man who owned and conducted a chain of saloons in connection with quarters for prostitutes. The wife knew nothing of her husband's business, and when one winter's night she discovered it, she came barefooted, clothed only in her night clothes, through the snow to my basement office, where I slept.

I took the shocked and shivering lady into bed with me. In the morning I called an ambulance and took her to the hospital, for she was in a state of truth-shock, quite as serious as shell-shock. The frantic husband was kept away for two weeks, during which time I was the go-between. The outcome was the wife's return, after the husband had disposed of his dives and purchased a leather-goods business. Happiness was completely restored, and the triumphant wife frequently visited, and sat for hours in the new store, which was successful in every way except that it crept daily deeper into the red. The husband, who was so successful in herding the black sheep of society, was fleeced by the white flock, and in order to keep the leather store looking prosperous, resorted to dipping surreptitiously into the old business. The leather-goods shop was a perfect camouflage for a long time. But a disastrous crash came.

Late one evening the patient's butler came for me in great excitement, and when I entered the sumptuous apartment, I saw on the couch a vision of loveliness—her troubles ended—asleep in death. A chloroform bottle on the floor told the story.

It was a long time before we reached the husband, but when he arrived and saw his wife, he fell prone on the floor, face downward, his high hat rolling in one direction and his cane in another.

In this way she innocently killed him, for from that moment his interest in life ceased. He withdrew, and lived alone in a single room until death came as a reward for loyalty to a great love.

My eye loves to rest on two camphor-wood chests. They are cunningly carved by the artful hands of the generous and honorable Chinese, and filled with memories of a year of life and work in the Orient. The most beautiful one of these chests I nearly missed, by a slip of the tongue. We had paid five dollars for the smaller one, carved by the prisoners in Nanchang, and had sent it to the steamship offices in Shanghai, where it escaped destruction in the earthquake.

About five years after returning from China, Alice remarked, "I don't see why I didn't get two of those chests."

I consoled her, "I will write to Dr. Ida Kahn, and have her send another."

At once I mailed a check for twenty-five dollars to Dr. Kahn, and requested her to duplicate the chest we had bought in Nanchang, and to keep any surplus money for her mission. We heard nothing from our order for nearly a year, when we received a summons to the customhouse in Chicago, to pay duty on a chest that had arrived from China. I repaired at once to the customhouse with my papers, and found the officer on duty very attentive. "This is quite a job, with many papers to sign. Make yourself comfortable, and I will speed it up as much as possible."

Every few moments he beckoned me to come and sign some schedule until finally he asked me a question. "Could this by chance be an antique?"

I was always so chatty on China that instead of saying, "No," which was all I really knew about the chest, I poured out this bit of information. "Oh, my no, that chest was made and carved by prisoners in Nanchang, China.

He looked so grave that I stopped talking, and he retired, to return shortly with the news, "I'm so sorry, but there is a United States commerce regulation that forces us to return the chest to China, on the ground that it was made by convict labor."

I have often had to make rapid surgical decisions, but now I

311

realized that I must not even appear to think, if I was to save that chest for Alice. I tried to look guileless instead of guilty. With assurance and as much surprise as I could muster, I offered an explanation. "I told you it was made by parishioners."

He gasped, "Excuse me; my mistake," and at once brought the clearance papers. We had no further conversation on the subject, and that chest, which was much larger and handsomer than the other, has been a closed subject. I have never tried to find out who made it, or where it was made, for I prefer to think that accidentally I did not lie to the gracious customs officer.

Every time I leave or enter the farmhouse I pass two six-hundred-pound carved stone lions, one on each side of the front entrance. This was another afterthought. We had greatly admired the many stone lions that we saw in China, and one day Alice expressed a wish. "I do so long for a pair of those Chinese lions that we saw on each side of every entrance in China."

I made my standard response, "The missionaries will send them if I write." Year after year I wrote, first to one and then to another, but no response ever came. Then I met Dr. Alice Barlow Brown, in Chicago on furlough from work in China.

She had been on my circuit surgical service when she was engaged in a large general practice in Winnetka, Illinois, and during World War I, under the auspices of the American Women's Hospitals of the American Medical Women's Association and the Red Cross, was commissioned to work with children in Paris. When she returned from her war service, everything in America seemed to her overfed, even obese, and she longed for engrossing work in lean and barren fields that were imperative in their need for medical help. China attracted her, and for the last more than twenty years she has been health officer in the Yencheng Women's College, besides organizer of a rural midwifery clinic and service near Peking. Recently, to the delight of her friends, she returned on one of those merciful trips of the Gripsholm, after spending six months in a concentration camp.

I begged Dr. Brown to buy and send me a pair of Chinese lions, and gave her a check for twenty-five dollars. After returning, she wrote me that she could get a pair for the amount of the check, but for fifty dollars she could get a handsome pair two and one-half feet high.

I sent a check by clipper mail, and it was not long before I was in receipt of a bill for the transportation of the stone lions. From China to San Francisco the cost was seven dollars and fifty cents, but from San Francisco to Chicago the freight bill was over a hundred and sixty dollars. Education is always more or less expensive, and I had to pay for my ignorance of freight rates.

If the stone lions had been shipped as cemetery pieces, it would have cost only a little over thirty dollars, but they had been classified as sculpture. Finally I made a settlement, paying sixty dollars, garden-ornament rate.

Our Ming lions, three hundred years old, give to the old millstone that lies between them at the front-door entrance a modern look, for its age is only one hundred and twenty-five years—the whole time of the history of Stony Creek.

The fireplace in the library has a jamb that is one story and a half high, and is fed with man-sized logs. Sparks from the blazing fire are restrained by a wire screen that Alice ordered from an art firm in Texas. The screen is in three sections. The center, the largest, executed in artistic ironwork, is a picture of Mount Moriah, Stony Creek's big hill, with pines waving and birds soaring over its top. The panels on the sides are in the spirit of the Chinese iron pictures. One side depicts Father, pick in hand, in 1851 in California; and on the other, Mother, an octogenarian, standing as erect as the tall silo on her right, with her apron billowing in the wind.

Every year on Christmas Eve we gather around the glowing grate and its screen, silhouetting Mother with her sturdy reserve, and Father with his jolly cheer. We pile our gifts on a long, backless settee in front of the fireplace. Seventy-five years ago this settee was used for a game that we called "bag of wheat."

The walnut flooring in the library was taken from Uncle Nathaniel Millerd's house, the first frame one built in Stony Creek. It is still standing, colonial in architecture, and literally built around a big central chimney. Many years after the builder had died, one of his relatives, who was a little confused in his mind, disappeared. When he was missed a search was instituted; the mill pond was drained; the woods were tramped; the wells emptied; the search spread for miles around Stony Creek, but the whereabouts of the feather-brained fugitive was not revealed. When the cold fall weather suggested the necessity for fires, the long-lost man appeared one morning at the breakfast table. He had hidden in the commodious chimney for several months, coming out only at night to forage for food.

The small red-marble clock in the kitchen strikes so rapidly that I would lose count if the cuckoo did not precede it with its slow, judicial cadence. The marble clock was the gift of a skilled nurse who struggled with invalidism through her course in Bellevue Hospital, New York City, and later in her superintendency of nurses in the New England Hospital for Women and Children. After I had been practicing in Chicago, she came to me in despair over her physical condition. I discovered the cause and operated on her. With restored health she accepted the entire charge of Red Cross work in the South, and acquitted herself so splendidly that the Red Cross presented her with a gold ring set with a large ruby.

When the marble clock becomes silent, the old clock whose weights Sarah winds up every night adds its hesitating, clanging strokes. This clock was found in the house where mother was married in 1854. For years it had been lost in the attic, but now under Sarah's care keeps excellent time.

On the piano in the library is a loving cup, now thirty years old, the thought of Dr. Alice Wynekoop. For many years I scarcely noticed it, but for the past ten years I have never passed it without offering a timid prayer for her.

As a child I had watched the stallion from the loft of the horse-barn that is the foundation of the library; I had toddled across its walnut floors; I had warmed myself, sitting on the hearth made of century-old, handmade, square bricks. Every nook and corner had something of my life.

24

GREAT-GREAT-GRANDFATHER LIVES ON

FROM EARLY CHILDHOOD, my ambition had been to please my father, to hear him say, "That's right. Make them hunt their holes; let them know there's a God in Israel." After his death the breaking of all these connecting threads consumed years, but while this dissolution was taking place, I was unconsciously replacing them with the warp and woof of a responsibility to future generations, through the instrumentality of my niece, Sarah.

Even before her birth I sewed into her layette the anticipated joys of a baby niece. At the age of six months she nearly died of double pneumonia. For three days I wept unceasingly, while assuring Alice that I had not given up hope, but that I could not waste my energy controlling emotions. Through Sarah, Christmas took on the light of the Star of Bethlehem.

She was four when her father died and my ambition swelled to be a father to her. To be a mother is a peculiarly hallowed relation not to be assumed casually, but the role of father is a more material tie, involving the dispensing of praise and privileges—and the payment of bills.

I had been playing Papa for two years when Sarah was suddenly attacked with a disease that the medical profession does not even yet understand, and for which no cure has been discovered. The only symptom of this rare, strange disease was thirst—an amazing thirst. Physician after physician diagnosed the trouble as Diabetes Insipidus, but none suggested treatment.

I took Sarah and Alice with me when I made my calls, and with a tiny commode and a large bottle of water in the buggy, we rode for hours every day, wondering what we could do for Sarah, and what the end might be.

On one of these days we passed a handsome gray-haired man with chiselled features, driving a Goddard buggy something like ours. Alice sighed, "How I wish we could have an old physician, like that beautiful man we just passed, take a look at Sarah."

I said, "Why, that was Dr. Quine. We can have him, I'm sure."

As soon as we reached home, I telephoned him. He and Sarah were friends at once as he advised not to restrict her drinking. He suggested that we have a blood examination, for strangely enough, we had not had one, although we had had almost every other laboratory test. He remarked with a mischievous look, "Have them examine the blood for malaria."

"Do you think she has malaria?" I asked.

"Oh, no," he chuckled. "But it is nice to have something to look for, when you are looking."

I tried to make Dr. Quine suggest a man to make the blood examination, but he insisted that no matter who made it, other pathologists would not concur. We settled on Dr. Klebs of Klebs-Loeffler bacillus fame, and when the report came, sure enough, the blood showed malaria! As Dr. Quine had predicted, no doctor would accept the report unless the laboratory he recommended made the diagnosis. Accordingly, we went from one laboratory to another, but from each came a positive diagnosis of malarial infection.

Dr. Quine now had a treatment, and suggested that Alice take Sarah to California, an antimalarial climate, and remain there until the blood showed no malaria, although Sarah had no symptoms of malaria—no fever, and no chills.

Moreover, we needed to make haste, for it was already December. Alice had promised Sarah that if we went, we would not leave Chicago until after Christmas, but realizing that it would be much easier traveling before Christmas, and a better time for me to be away from my practice, I asked Alice, "What is the use of having Christmas come on the twenty-fifth of December every year? This year it is going to come on the twelfth!"

She shook her head dubiously, but laughed, and though the ghost of a lie was repulsive to her, agreed to the new Christmas date and made plans to that effect.

To promote the new date, I made frequent remarks, "Just ten days before Christmas. Only a week before Christmas." The ruse went over splendidly, and the only explanation we had to make was why we had another Christmas in Pasadena. By explaining the difference in time between Chicago and California, the mystery was solved satisfactorily to the child's mind.

After three years' residence on the Pacific coast the malaria disappeared from the blood, but Sarah's diabetes did not abate. Even so, she became well enough to return to Chicago.

Up to the time Sarah entered school, and afterwards during summer vacations, she stayed with Alice on the farm that she loved so much that she used to say, "I don't want to go back to Chicago, where nothing ever happens. I want to stay on the farm, where something happens every minute."

Alice and I should have recognized Sarah's vocational aptitude for farming, that she had displayed when a tiny tot. When she was about four years old, we had been watching her as she returned from the barns. She wore blue overalls, the legs of which were tucked into her high rubber boots. Every step she took was as long as her short legs allowed, and gave the appearance of a small wooden soldier with its stiff mechanical movements. We restrained our laughter when she entered the room and laid down her currycombs and brushes. "Sarah, look at those boots! Go into the woodshed and clean them!"

As Sarah trudged out of the farmhouse living room without a word of surprise or explanation, no one guessed that her own pudgy hands had daubed on the manure to imitate the smell of the hired men, for whom she had profound admiration.

Alice and I must have had eyes that see not, for such exhibitions of her talent for farming were of daily occurrence. It was not until she was on the eve of graduating from the University of Chicago that she disclosed the allurement that farm life had for her, and her ambitions.

Alice and I had a big jolt when Sarah remarked, "Next fall I will begin my premedic course, and after I have my medical education, I will practice until I have earned enough money to buy a farm. How long do you think it will take?"

We gasped, and in unison burst out, "So that is what you want to do—farm?"

"Oh, yes!" She turned to her mother. "But I thought you and Gub wanted me to study medicine."

"Farming is not what it was when Grandfather ran the farm," I explained. "In these times a farmer should be a graduate of an agricultural college."

"May I?" She was all eagerness.

That precipitated the solution.

The next week I went with Sarah to Madison, Wisconsin, where she matriculated for the summer term in the Agricultural Department of the University of Wisconsin, to work for an M.S. degree, majoring in Animal Husbandry.

After she received her M.S. degree, Professor Cole, under whom she had been working, was anxious for her to remain and take a Ph.D. degree in Genetics, but when she enrolled for this high degree, she had no idea that it would require five years. The delay in receiving her degree was occasioned by World War I. When the student in charge of pigeon research enlisted, the pigeons were turned over to Sarah. The student with guinea-pig experiments followed, and Sarah was put in charge of the guinea pigs. Students continued to leave, one after another, and their research animals were consigned to Sarah. Professor Cole would say, "You can have any of the younger boys to help, but we shall have to depend upon you to keep our problems going."

When Sarah was in touch with all departments of animal study—mice, pigeons, guinea pigs, dogs, sheep, cows and horses

—Professor Cole came to her with the information, "I may be called to Washington for an indefinite period, and may have to leave the department in your care."

Personally, I believe that such an experience is an opportunity of a lifetime and worth a dozen degrees, but it made the taking of her Ph.D. degree impossible before June, 1921.

Mother was in her ninety-first year when Sarah took this advanced degree, but was anxious to go to Madison for the event. Unfortunately she became ill and was unable to take the trip. Sarah came home for a week end the week before graduation. Mother was delighted because she wanted to give Sarah a graduation present of a deed to our farm in Michigan which had been ceded to Great-grandfather by President Monroe.

She asked Sarah to dress up and march around the room before receiving her gift. Sarah thought it a joke but marched till her grandmother was quite satisfied. Then she knelt by her grandmother's bed and was given the deed to the farm. Sitting on the floor with her cheek buried in the palm that for almost a century had guarded the traditions of the Taylor family, the poor child was completely overcome. While I was thanking God for the privilege of having helped to save a baby's life so many years ago, Sarah was accepting the deed to those acres as a solemn trust and obligation.

Sarah and her grandmother were very close to each other, and I think Sarah had a stronger family feeling than any other descendant of the ten children and the twenty-six grandchildren that her great-great-grandfather had brought to Stony Creek.

Mother had spent every summer, except the one when we were in Europe, on the farm. Sarah had joined her until prevented by the study of agriculture at Madison, Wisconsin. Chicago had been Mother's winter home and she had been very happy to be with her girls.

Even after her ninetieth birthday she was self-reliant, able to care for herself, and enjoy a movie several times a week. Consequently, when she fell ill, it seemed strange to all of us to be carrying trays of food to her. We tried to accustom ourselves to the thought that she might never recover and gradually this fact became plain for us. She did not suffer except that it was difficult for her to breathe.

She had been confined to her bed only two weeks when, as Father had done twenty-five years before, she fell into coma, and in a few days ceased her efforts to breathe.

We took her from our Chicago home back to the farmhouse in Stony Creek, that had been her home since 1830.

On the 27th of June, 1921, the ninety-eighth June of the Taylor migration, the village flag flew at half-mast—this flag that her hands had helped raise and dedicate in the last war. She had seen three wars, but no one had roused her more than this last one. Her eyes could look back from these days of electricity to those when tallow dips were the only light, and many candles had her hands moulded. From oxcart to the automobile, from tallow candles to electric light, she had passed with never a thought or look backward, for to her, old days were never the best ones; she loved progress, and to the very last kept abreast of the times.

For three days the neighbors came and went, many sitting by the hour, watching her peaceful face. There was a sort of sanctity in her presence too great for display of grief. In life she had refined all within her world—so it was in death.

Alice and I realized that as a farmer Sarah would lead a healthful outdoor life, and we thought that the responsibilities of a farmer would be less demanding than the strain and worry of a physician. This attitude demonstrated how little we who had been brought up on a farm understood farming.

It may have been a trait inherited from some of her Dutch-English-Welsh ancestors, for Sarah would never buy an automobile, farm equipment, or animals until she thought such expenditures were warranted.

In 1924 she started with chickens, and assumed their entire care. When I saw her carrying great pails of water and sacks of feed, even cleaning chicken coops, it was hard to believe that she was making the best use of all the degrees she had acquired.

She was, however, determined to know her business from the ground up, and never vacillated from this position.

As soon as Sarah had a firm hold on the chicken business, she employed a man for manual work, and in the fall of 1927 took over the management of the farm, the raising of the crops and the production of certified milk. With unflagging patience and persistent effort, she has coaxed bumper crops from the land, and rehabilitated Stony Creek. I was as proud as Mother's peacock, watching Sarah and Alice create a splendid estate out of the old run-down farm.

Soon after Sarah started her poultry department, the chickens died by the dozens, of coccydiosis. As a preventive, I suggested putting iodine into the drinking water, and a short time after she began using it, I could hardly believe my senses when I saw instead of white, a flock of yellow leghorns. Every feather had turned a brilliant yellow.

When Sarah told me of an umbilical hernia in a valuable calf, I bought bolts of adhesive tape and bandaged it so successfully that I had the pleasure of seeing the calf cured.

Cows have a dramatic disease called puerperal paresis, in which a newly freshened cow appears to be suddenly paralyzed in her hind legs, sinks to the ground, becoming comatose, and if not cared for, dies. A remedy for this condition is to inject air through the teats until the udder is fully distended. Almost before this treatment has been completed, the cow regains consciousness, gets up, and begins chewing her cud.

This treatment for the puerperal paresis in cows gave me an idea for controlling the high blood pressure that precedes puerperal toxemia and convulsions in the expectant mother. As soon as a slight rise in blood pressure is discovered in the pregnant woman, I express the secretion from her breasts and teach her to do the same, three or four times a day. Through this practice alone, I frequently reduce a rising blood pressure in pregnancy to normal limits.

The prevention of goiter in calves, by giving the cows iodized salt, has encouraged me to give iodine to expectant mothers, and to advise them to give some iodine preparation to the growing child at stated periods during the year.

When it became noised about Stony Creek that I was coming more or less regularly, many people in the community asked to consult me regarding their health. This resulted in my seeing patients at the farm bimonthly, that is, every other Sunday morning, and operating in Detroit or Pontiac on the Saturday before.

My Stony Creek practice involved a bus ride of six hundred miles round trip from Chicago, and an automobile ride of a hundred miles or more, shuttling back and forth between Detroit and the farm in order to devote two Saturdays each month to operating, and two Sunday mornings to seeing patients.

Pneumonia, in the fall of 1939, followed in July, 1940, by a virulent streptococcic infection of my hand, with loss of my left index finger, and a gangrenous appendix in October of the same year, forced me to discontinue, after fifteen years, my Stony Creek Sunday morning office and my Saturday operations in Detroit and Pontiac. In spite of this, the medical service rendered to the community of my birth resulted in attracting Dr. Elizabeth Stone, an especially well-equipped medical woman, to begin practice in a nearby town, where the public, through my efforts, had become "woman-doctor minded".

As I had built up an office and surgical practice in Stony Creek to ensure my future happiness by having, when I left Chicago, a full-fledged practice to continue, instead of retiring—so Sarah has carried out similar protective measures by not putting all of her eggs in one basket. She has a fifteen-hundred-bird-capacity poultry plant besides her dairy where she raises purebred Holstein-Fresian cattle, selling many animals every year. Her animals have taken so many prizes at state and county agricultural fairs that her office is decorated with a frieze of champion and grand champion ribbons. Almost every year she is chosen by the Michigan State Holstein-Fresian Association as a delegate to the national convention. She has also served as president of that association.

1942 brought Sarah a harvest of honors. In the spring the

National Holstein-Fresian Association, after judging our herd, admitted it to Progressive Breeders' Registry. Sarah is the only lady breeder to receive that distinction. In the summer she received the ribbons for Premier Breeder at the Waterloo Dairy Cattle Congress, a national show where forty-six herds were exhibited. Finally, she was given a high mark of public confidence when she was elected to the Board of the Michigan State College of Agriculture at East Lansing. For many years she has been a Master Farmer.

No father has ever gloated more over the laurels bestowed upon his offspring than I, over Sarah's successes in farming. Even when she was small she registered her feeling about me by announcing, "My, but I was lucky that my father died."

"Why, Sarah!" Alice spoke with disapproval. "What has your aunt or I ever said to make you speak like that?"

Sarah was firm. "All right, but he would never have done for me all the things that Gub has."

Instead of worrying about the uncontrollable fluctuations in the certified milk market, three years ago Sarah built a farm store for the distribution of her farm products at firsthand. It is located across the road from the farmhouse, in the village of Stony Creek, one mile from an arterial highway. For nearly one hundred years a small general store had been in operation on this site; but during the past thirty years the store had been in the earth-to-earth-ashes-to-ashes category.

When Sarah learned that is was about to be converted into a beer hall, she bought the property and has made as much a show place of it as Alice has made of our house and grounds.

Sarah named the store The Sign of the Black and White Cow and a colonial style board swinging from the corner of the building proclaims it. Its cobblestone corner approach, the iron horsehead hitching posts, the high field-stone fireplace, the wagon wheel set with candles for lighting, the hundred-year-old counters, the boarded walls and ceiling—all make it worth while to stray from the highway.

Here the city feeders flock for butter, cream, cottage cheese, buttermilk, all grades of fresh eggs, milk (certified, vitamin D certified, homogenized certified, or natural soft-curd certified), broilers, turkeys in season—all Sarah's farm products.

To serve her community she sells for a small commission any product of good quality, originating in the community. In this manner her stock includes homemade bread, cakes and cookies, jams, jellies, canned fruit, stone-ground flour of all kinds, honey, maple sugar, homemade candy, nuts, fresh fruit and vegetables in season, and every description of handiwork.

Hikers from Detroit, classes of school children from neighboring towns, clubs of young people and adults, find that a trip to the farm, with a visit to the barns and chicken houses, a peep around the charming village, and a stop at the store where they can get a standing lunch of milk and cookies or chicken salad sandwiches, provides a unique and enjoyable outing.

In connection with, and at one side of the store, is the farm office where a bookkeeper is always laboring to keep abreast of bills, cow pedigrees, store accounts and office records. It is here that Sarah meets the score of men employed on the farm and those who come on business.

Through Sarah I have learned that farming is as exacting in its demands as medicine, if not more so; that it requires as much, or more, preparation; that it is as necessary and vital a service to humanity; and that its rewards in the joy of daily performance and the hope of gaining, as Sarah expresses it, "perfection through efficiency", are the same.

Being a father to Sarah gave to my life a supreme motive, for it was Sarah whose life has been knitted into the pattern of my days from the time when I carefully counted and set up stitches, until now when I am at the end, narrowing off.

SIGNAL LIVES:
Autobiographies of American Women

An Arno Press Collection

Antin, Mary. **The Promised Land,** 1969

Atherton, Gertrude Franklin [Horn]. **Adventures of a Novelist,** 1932

Bacon, Albion Fellows. **Beauty for Ashes,** 1914

Bailey, Abigail. **Memoirs of Mrs. Abigail Bailey who had been the Wife of Major Asa Bailey Formerly of Landhoff (N.H.),** 1815

Barr, Amelia E.H. **All The Days of my Life,** 1913

Barton, Clara. **The Story of my Childhood,** 1924

Belmont, Eleanor Robson. **The Fabric of Memory,** 1957

Boyle, Sarah Patton. **The Desegregated Heart,** 1962

Brown, Harriet Connor. **Grandmother Brown's Hundred Years,** 1929

Burnett, Frances Hodgson. **The One I Know Best of All,** 1893

Carson, Mrs. Ann. **The Memoirs of the Celebrated and Beautiful Mrs. Ann Carson, Daughter of an Officer of the U.S. Navy and Wife of Another, Whose Life Terminated in the Philadelphia Prison,** 1838

Churchill, Caroline Nichols. **Active Footsteps,** 1909

Cleghorn, Sarah N. **Threescore,** 1936

[Dall, Caroline H.W.]. **Alongside,** 1900

Daviess, Maria Thompson. **Seven Times Seven,** 1924

Dorr, Rheta Child. **A Woman of Fifty,** 1924

[Dumond], Annie H. Nelles. **The Life of a Book Agent,** 1868

Eaton, [Margaret O'Neale]. **The Autobiography of Peggy Eaton,** 1932

Farrar, Mrs. John [Elizabeth Rotch]. **Recollections of Seventy Years,** 1866

Felton, Rebeca Latimer. **Country Life in Georgia in the Days of my Youth,** 1919

Garden, Mary and Louis Biancolli. **Mary Garden's Story,** 1951

Gildersleeve, Virginia Crocheron. **Many a Good Crusade,** 1954

Gilson, Mary Barnett. **What's Past is Prologue,** 1940

Hurst, Fannie. **Anatomy of Me,** 1958

Jacobs-Bond, Carrie. **The Roads of Melody,** 1927

Jelliffe, Belinda. **For Dear Life,** 1936

Jones, Amanda T. **A Psychic Autobiography,** 1910

Logan, Kate Virginia Cox. **My Confederate Girlhood,** 1932

Longworth, Alice Roosevelt. **Crowded Hours,** 1933

MacDougall, Alice Foote. **The Autobiography of a Business Woman,** 1928

Madeleine. 1919

Meyer, Agnes E. **Out of These Roots,** 1953

Odlum, Hortense. **A Woman's Place,** 1939

Potter, Eliza. **A Hairdresser's Experience in High Life,** 1859

Rinehart, Mary Roberts. **My Story,** 1948

[Ritchie], Anna Cora Mowatt. **Autobiography of an Actress,** 1854

Robinson, Josephine DeMott. **The Circus Lady,** 1925

Roe, Mrs. Elizabeth A. **Recollections of Frontier Life,** 1885

Sanders, Sue. **Our Common Herd,** 1939

Sangster, Margaret E. **An Autobiography,** 1909

Sherwood, M[ary] E[lizabeth]. **An Epistle to Posterity,** 1897

Sigourney, Mrs. L[ydia] H. **Letters of Life,** 1866

Smith, Elizabeth Oakes [Prince]. **Selections from the Autobiography of Elizabeth Oakes Smith,** 1924

[Terhune], Mary V.H. **Marion Harland's Autobiography,** 1910

Terrell, Mary Church. **A Colored Woman in a White World,** 1940

Ueland, Brenda. **Me,** 1939

Van Hoosen, Bertha. **Petticoat Surgeon,** 1947

Vorse, Mary Heaton. **A Footnote to Folly,** 1935

[Ward], Elizabeth Stuart Phelps. **Chapters from a Life,** 1896

Wilcox, Ella Wheeler. **The Worlds and I,** 1896

Wilson, Edith Bolling. **My Memoir,** 1938